Sperm Tales

An Informative Guide Through the Challenges of Infertility

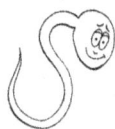

Sperm Tales

An Informative Guide Through the Challenges of Infertility

Lynn M. Collins

Collins, Lynn, M.

Sperm Tales / Lynn M. Collins—1st. ed.

ISBN 978-0-9965203-0-0

Dedication

This book is dedicated to women who are infertile and may be in a program; and to those who are having difficulty understanding and under a lot of stress. I hope *Sperm Tales* can take your hand and get you through the tough times and the good times.

I feel confident that *Sperm Tales* will help you understand what your nurse and specialist are saying to you and your partner. And if there are decisions to be made, I hope the book will help make those decisions easier. I want *Sperm Tales* to take the stress away (with the help of some yoga classes or acupuncture and Reiki). I want women to feel empowered and strong, but at the same time not afraid to cry. I know *Sperm Tales* will put infertility in the right perspective with less stress so you can say, "I'm doing this!" You'll have that baby.

This book is also for young women in new careers, working hard and loving it! I wrote *Sperm Tales* to help you think about your fertility and realize the time may come when you need help and add this to your plan. We as women have much on our plate and your fertile years can slip away quickly. But I hope *Sperm Tales* will help you organize your life.

Contents

Introduction

Infertility is a medical problem defined as the failure of a couple to conceive a child after one year of unprotected sexual intercourse, or the inability to carry a pregnancy to live birth. According to the American Society for Reproductive Medicine (ASRM), infertility affects about 6.1 million people in the United States, which is about 10 percent of the reproductive age population.

Increasingly people are turning to physicians who specialize in Assisted Reproductive Technologies (ART) to address these problems. In 1981 only a single baby was born in the U.S. by means of ART. In contrast, by 2009, ART reported over 146,000 cycles to the Center for Disease Control (CDC) resulting in 45,870 live births.[1]

Both men and women can be infertile. According to the ASRM, one third of the time the diagnosis is due to female infertility; one third of the time it is linked to male infertility; the remaining one third is due to a combination of factors from both partners. In approximately 20 percent of cases, the cause of a couple's infertility cannot be determined.

I have managed an infertility laboratory for over 12 years and have been closely involved with physicians and nurses on a day-to-day basis, as well as with the couples participating in the program. Over the years I have intimately engaged both partners and their respective experiences, including couples who struggled intensively with this process and those who breezed through it without major complications or issues. Even those who seem to have very little difficulty still crave information related to infertility and the process of tackling it. I recently surveyed 75 couples within the program asking if they thought it would be helpful to have a book about infertility and its challenges. They were unanimous in their consent that such a book would benefit them and more, they wanted to know where they could buy a copy. I myself looked for resources in the library and on the internet to see what was out there to help these couples. I found only a few references, and those seemed to me to be too scientific and obtuse for anyone to understand unless they are a physician or nurse. At that point I realized the acute need to write a layperson's book for confused and often struggling couples who desire to know more about infertility, the process, and their options.

To some extent, societal changes and trends have driven the evolution of infertility practices and the ongoing need for it. Most of our mothers' generation had their children during the years of their twenties, when women are most fertile. The women of today have more options, opportunities and, in some cases, necessity to have a career. In most cases the rising costs of living creates the need for a double income in order to maintain even a modest standard of living. That has become the norm in our culture.

Other factors as well drive the need for ART. Women today tend to pursue their careers and goals *before* they have children yet all the while the biological clock is ticking away. Often divorced couples who remarry desire to start a family with the second partner. Same-sex couples want to have a family. Many single women who haven't found the right man often look to ART to have a child independently. In other instances, some couples have no problems getting pregnant, but can't carry the baby to full term and lose the pregnancy. Other couples have recurrent miscarriages (defined as three or more consecutive losses). Thus, it has come to pass that many couples in a variety of circumstances seek help from an infertility clinic. The downside to the advance in this field is that it could, in some instances render a false sense of assurance that having a child won't be a problem and so some put it off, sometimes for decades, waiting to start trying after their body's most fertile years have peaked and are in decline. It is my hope in this book to render sound and practical advice to any person or couple desiring to start a family, how to decide when, and what to do if difficulty conceiving ensues.

Infertility is a personal and private part of a couple's life. The desire to have a child and the inability to do so can create a great deal of emotional stress in even the best relationship. There are many unanswered questions couples face when beginning an infertility program and the infertility puzzle has multiple pieces. Some couples have little knowledge of the emotional, physical, and financial impact the process will impose on their lives. Most couples are informed on some of the techniques involved, but need to know specifics about how each technique relates to their specific situation. Every couple's circumstance is unique and presents different issues that must be addressed on an individual basis.

I cannot stress enough the importance of communication when discussing the topic of infertility. For some, talking about these delicate matters comes easily, while others have much difficulty. From the start it is helpful for you to get comfortable, let go of your inhibitions, and keep an open mind. Discussion about such topics as sex, intercourse, and masturbation is common and the use of the term "sperm" is commonplace. Most people feel vulnerable and embarrassed when these matters are discussed. It may take time to feel safe before opening up honestly and being able to converse in this way with your infertility specialist. Don't worry. Those of us in the field have all seen and heard all sorts of things. We are there to help you.

The actual title of the Infertility Specialist is called a Reproductive Endocrinologist (RE). The RE is a physician who is trained in reproductive medicine addressing hormonal functioning as it pertains to reproduction as well as infertility. He or she is also trained in Obstetrics and Gynecology (OB-GYN). During the book, as I frequently refer to the RE, I'll use the term interchangeably with "specialist." See! You are starting to learn the infertility lingo.

It will be essential for you to ask questions and listen. You are going to be absorbing a lot of information. If you are not sure about something you are being told or have read about, then ask your doctor or nurse. Beyond that, keep in mind that this is a team effort and there are specific aspects of it that you, as a couple, must assume. It is important that all instructions given to you be followed as directed by your nursing team. Keep this in mind and do your part. It will help everyone involved.

Finally, in addition to providing the necessary information to help you anticipate in the process, one of my special goals in this book is to make couples laugh. I want to make this journey fun, at least in some small way. To that end, I want you to meet a friend who will help us along this journey. His name is Spanky. He came to me on one of my birthdays when a fellow nurse gave me a plastic toy sperm with pink eyes and a wrapped condom sticking out of his mouth. I held a contest to name it and we shared hilarity as more people became involved, including our infertility patients. Among the many entries from staff and patients, the patients made the final decision calling him Spanky, who now sits on a desk and has become the clinic's mascot. Over the course of the many years working in the clinic I have kept a small notebook in which I wrote funny comments I heard from patients. Throughout the book Spanky will interject some of these humorous asides. He will serve to remind us that there are times during this process when things come up and you simply have to laugh. Spanky will help you do this. So let us begin this journey together!

Chapter 1
When Should I Have My Baby?

Confusion and lack of understanding about the basic aspects of this critical decision pervade the early stages of this journey.

I read an article in *Newsweek* in 2001[2] focusing on different women who pondered when they wanted to start their families, most of whom chose to put it off for several years. Some were at the height of their careers; others were traveling or going to graduate school. They had no social life and felt that this wasn't the right time to have children. One woman who was in medical school knew she was pushing the biological time clock. Even so, she felt that the advancement in technology would help her conceive by the time she was ready. Another woman found her "Mr. Right" at the age of 42 and decided then she wanted to start her family. (*If movie stars can get pregnant at 40, why can't I?*) Over the next few years this woman and her husband tried to conceive naturally with no success. They went to a fertility specialist and, in time, were able to conceive, but then miscarried. She was devastated. She could not have imagined she would have such a problem conceiving. She asked herself, "What did

I do? Did I wait too long to start trying?" Worse, she had spent over $3,000 for the first month of injectable medications.

The general misunderstandings and misguided assumptions about the process are often made worse by the hesitancy of some doctors to mention the topic to their younger patients. The above-mentioned *Newsweek* article highlights that many physicians choose not to bring up fertility plans to women under 35 unless the patient herself initiates it. The reasons for this include the idea that some doctors assume that women are aware of the issues related to their fertility or they fear that if it's brought up it might cause them distress or encourage them to make a premature decision to have a child before they are ready. As it is, when a woman visits her OB-GYN for the first time the physician usually will ask if the patient is sexually active and if she is using birth control.

Times have changed. The first "test tube baby"—conceived by In Vitro Fertilization (IVF)—was born in July of 1978. At that time ART procedures had undergone long drawn-out experimental stages and approval of such technology from the Federal Drug Administration (FDA) involved a lengthy process. Since then, however, women are delaying childbearing as never before: the rate of first births for women in their thirties and forties has quadrupled since 1970.[3] At the same time, rates of women in their early twenties have dropped by a third. A woman is born with a limited number of eggs, which gradually get ovulated or die off as she ages. The quality of the older eggs diminishes, lessoning the chance of fertilization.

Women are more fertile in their twenties than the thirties and forties. The chances of conceiving for women in the later years drops by five to ten per cent per year.

These trends portend challenges for older couples wanting children and for developing ongoing IVF technologies to keep up with these trends.

Has much changed since the article in *Newsweek*?

I asked this question to a group of young people:

At what age do you think a woman's fertility diminishes and she'll need to seek help from an infertility specialist?[4]

Their answers are noted below. The first column represents the age of the women asked the question and the second column is their answer. The third column is the age of the males asked the same question and the fourth column is their answer. For example, the first woman I asked was 36 years of age and her answer was that woman would start seeking help at the age of 60.

(For the sake of continuity the entire study is rendered on the following page.)

Lynn M. Collins

Infertility Age Survey

Females Asked		Males Asked	
Age:	Answer	Age:	Answer
36	60	38	40
24	45	35	40
25	50	23	38
33	48	36	38
43	35	33	40
24	43	34	35
23	45	28	35
21	43	27	36
30	40	28	43
25	30	23	40
21	36	23	40
30	35	26	40
25	32	22	35
26	32	38	25
25	40	32	35

The answer to the question – *at what age do you think a woman's fertility diminishes and she'll need to seek help from an infertility specialist?* – is 35. This is the point at which fertility, for most women, drops significantly. A woman is most fertile between the ages of 18 and 25, with a small decline during the next 10 years. The decline becomes much more dramatic at the age of 35. Thus, women who are serious about having a family should actually seek advice and help before 35 years of age.[5] It is worth noting that, in the above survey, only one third of the answers marked the critical age at 35 years or less.

The TV show *60 Minutes* aired a program[6] that highlighted five successful women, their ages varying from late forties to early fifties, who had not had any children. Their careers had so consumed them that biological time clock had slipped away before they knew it.

They also interviewed five women in their freshman year at Harvard and asked them the same question I asked my group. The age they felt that women would seek help is in their fifties. They said with all the new procedures (In-Vitro Fertilization, IVF) and science available today would help women get pregnant. So, they concluded, they would just wait.

My informal survey, the five successful women highlighted in the *60 Minutes* program as well as the women interviewed from Harvard, demonstrate convincingly that many people, including highly educated ones, remain unaware of what age fertility drops precipitously and so jeopardized the ability to conceive. *Sperm Tales* is an attempt to help patients start an Infertility program on time and so heighten the chance for success, and also to educate young people to keep a clear head about this harsh reality as they plan their lives, families and careers.

It is critical that OB-GYNs talk to their patients up front and early on to make them aware of the age their fertility starts to diminish. My OB-GYN repeatedly said to me,

"Lynn you are getting close to 35 and your fertility will drop dramatically" and "what are you waiting for?"[7]

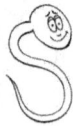 panky says:

"I have a low sperm count.
What can I do to get it up?"

Chapter 2
How To Choose a Fertility Center

Once a couple has determined that their situation warrants medical intervention or, at the very least, consultation, how do you choose where to go and who to see? The survey highlighted in the previous chapter notes that 35 years of age is the target number to aim for in making the decision to consult a specialist. In anticipation of this, couples should try for six months to conceive on their own. After that, if they are not successful, then the time has come to choose an expert to help navigate the next steps. Most couples should try for 12 months if the female is in her late 20s early 30s. After that, if not successful, then it's time to get help. If a female is aware that she is at risk of infertility because of irregular monthly periods, she should seek help when ready to start a family. Choosing an expert to help you get pregnant is one of the most important decisions you'll make.

Several questions that you should keep in mind when making this important decision include the following:

- How many years has the program been in operation?
- Does it have a good reputation?

- Does the center perform the IVF procedure at that clinic or at another location?
- Do they have an age limit for the female in the IVF program?

Beyond these, I've highlighted several other key points that need to be part of the process of decision-making.

Key points to keep in mind
Success Rate

Typically, when you start treatment you may start with Intra-Uterine Insemination (IUI) (to be discussed in detail later). In most cases patients will move onto Invitro Fertilization (IVF), so this is the process and the success rate the patient will want to focus upon.[8]

By law, every fertility clinic or hospital has to report their IVF success rates. The website for the Society for Assisted Reproductive Technologies (SART) (www.sart. org) provides all relevant statistics for any given center. These statistics include how many patients the clinic has treated and their age groups. The "live birth rate" will tell you how many women delivered a live baby through a particular center and not simply how many got pregnant. (Many women get pregnant in a clinic, but may have miscarried or a cycle could have been cancelled.)[9] All fertility centers include all results in the statistics. According to SART, the national average percentage of live births in 2010 for women under age of 35 was 41.7 percent. The live-birth success rate for those between the ages of 38 and 40 was 22.2 percent. This gives you a point of reference for helping you choose a center: look for a center with a live-birth success rate above the average.

Once you feel confident about a program or center, make a preliminary appointment with the specialist, together as a couple, to determine your comfort and confidence level. Infertility can be very stressful and there are going to be many ups and downs emotionally. So you want to be sure you feel comfortable and have the clear sense that this specialist cares for you. The clinic should be open seven days a week and you should be able to contact a nurse or specialist 24/7. (When I first interviewed for the infertility position, someone told me that I wouldn't need to work on weekends or holidays. Well, I found out that women don't pick just Monday thru Friday to ovulate!)

Emotional Support

During the course of infertility treatment, patients often express a sense of loss of control over their lives, especially when pregnancy does not come quickly. Infertility is a medical condition that affects every part of a person's life. It can make you question the way you feel about yourself, your relationship with others, and life in general. You may experience frustration and anger: *My friends and co-workers are getting pregnant, why aren't I?* Some patients keep their infertility a secret and choose not to let family members or friends know. All of these fine points in the process become a source of stress. And high stress levels can contribute to illness and exacerbate the problem. This makes it all the more important that the center offers infertility counseling and support groups. Even for those who choose to share the situation with family, friends and medical staff, may benefit from the assistance of professional counseling.[10]

To give you an idea of the stress level infertility imposes, one needs to look at the "Holmes and Rahe stress scale," which assigns a rating score reflecting the level of stress to people during certain events. Holmes and Rahe are psychiatrists and in 1967 reviewed over 5000 medical records so as to determine if stressful events in one's life can cause illness. Ranging from one to 100 the Social Readjustment Rating Scale (SRRS) lists a vacation as a 13; getting a major mortgage as 32; the death of a spouse as 100.[11] Infertility is also a life-changing event and ranks 39. So it is important to explore how—and if—the clinic a patient chooses accommodates the emotional needs for the patient.

The National Infertility Association, also known as RESOLVE, is a tremendous asset that every infertility couple should explore. Established in 1974, RESOLVE is a non-profit organization whose mission is to provide "timely, compassionate support and information to people who are experiencing infertility." RESOLVE's local support groups are led by therapists, peer groups, or others who have experienced infertility. The support groups, available throughout the United States, meet on a weekly or monthly basis and assure participants that you are not alone. You can learn much from these groups and it may help you to choose an infertility center. To find out if a support group is available in your area visit, http://www.

resolve.org/ and click under Local RESOLVE, to find out what region you belong to. Each region has its own web site, which has much information on infertility and will keep you updated about what's new.

Location

When choosing a center, keep in mind the location as it relates to your work or home. Once you begin a program you will make many visits there. It may be less stressful if you choose a center nearby. Some patients who lived in our area had initially chosen to go into a city to have their testing done. But once they realized they could get the same treatment closer to home they were thrilled. It changed their entire experience for the better. Imagine getting up before dawn to drive, say, upwards of 25 or 30 miles, waiting to have blood drawn and also an ultrasound, then turning around to go to work. This in itself is stressful. Then add the pressure of being late for work coupled with the turmoil of not wanting your employer to know your personal business. It is worth the time to check out all possibilities and seek to find one that is not too far afield from the location of your home and work.

Insurance and Treatment Parameters

It is the responsibility of the patient to find out what benefits are included in infertility coverage, including medications. Call your insurance company ahead of time and see what your options and limitations are for this. Infertility is very expensive and it's best to take charge and understand your coverage to avoid any surprises after a procedure indicating you owe money you didn't expect to have to pay.

Understanding insurance benefits can be confusing for many people when exploring infertility coverage, especially when it comes to deciphering the medical lingo that apply to these treatments. In most cases, those patients fortunate enough to have infertility coverage with their insurance plan are limited to a certain dollar amount or number of treatment cycles. A treatment cycle is considered any of the ART cycles, either Intra-Uterine Insemination (IUI) or In-Vitro Fertilization (IVF). It is important to obtain written confirmation of your exact benefits plan in order to make the most appropriate choices when exploring treatment options. For example, you could have very limited coverage, which may give you treatment for two or three attempts, so your RE may move you right into a more aggressive treatment plan from the beginning.

Ask the insurance company how they define "infertility." Be aware that there may be restrictions of the type of fertility specialist you can see and that in some cases a pre-authorization may be necessary. Ask about the limits to your coverage as they apply to what types of infertility treatment cycles and procedures. How many IUI cycles are you allowed? How many IVF cycles are you allowed? Are there prerequisites that need to be realized before the next step? Does the treatment include drug coverage? (The drug coverage is very important. A cycle on medications could cost up to $3,000.00 to $4,000.00 for a single cycle, which is a month.) Do they specify which pharmacies you are allowed to use to fill your medications? Some insurance companies will cover up to the diagnosis of infertility but nothing beyond that. This means they will cover what procedures are necessary to come to the diagnosis of infertility, but after that there is no coverage.

Below I've listed the main questions you'll want to ask:

- Is the initial consultation and diagnostic testing covered?
- Is Intrauterine Insemination (IUI), also called Artificial Insemination, covered?
- Is In-Vitro Fertilization (IVF) covered?
- Is there any coverage for the medications associated with these treatments (sometimes referred to as "injectables")?
- Are pre-existing conditions excluded? If so, what qualifies as pre-existing?
- Do we have to meet any special medical criteria to use the benefit?
- Is there a maximum benefit amount? Is it a dollar amount or a number of cycles? Is it annual or lifetime? What counts toward the maximum diagnostic testing, medications or just treatments?
- Are there deductibles, co-pays and/or co-insurance?
- Do we need a referral in order to see a fertility specialist?
- Do we need prior authorization for consultation, testing or treatment?[12]

To give you an idea of coverage and what is included,

31

below I've include the state of Massachusetts and their infertility coverage, which was initiated in 1987:

According to the Massachusetts infertility insurance law, health insurance companies and health mainte-nance organizations (HMOs) that cover pregnancy-relat-ed benefits must also provide coverage for the medically necessary expenses for infertility diagnosis and fertility treatment costs, including IVF costs. [13]

The law on fertility treatment insurance was amended in 2010 and redefined the definition of infertility as an in-dividual who is "unable to conceive or produce concep-tion" during a period of one year if the woman is under the age of 35. If the woman is over the age of 35, the period of time is only six months.

Infertility Insurance Limitations

According to the Massachusetts infertility insurance mandate, insurance companies are not required to pro-vide coverage for the following fertility treatments:

- Any experimental fertility treatment or procedure, until the procedure has been recognized as non-experimental by the Commissioner
- Surrogacy (an agreement between parties to carry a pregnancy for intended parents)
- Reversal of voluntary sterilization (reversal of va-sectomy or tubal ligation)
- Cryopreservation of eggs (egg freezing)

Does My State Cover Infertility Treatment?

In recent years certain states have introduced laws requiring certain providers to offer or cover specific fertility treatments. These laws are known as mandates. To date 15 states have enacted some form of infertility insurance mandate. Here is a list of the 15 states, Arkansas, California, Connecticut, Hawaii, Illinois, Louisiana, Maryland, Massachusetts, Montana, New Jersey, New York, Ohio, Rhode Island, Texas, and West Virginia.

Some patients work in a different state then where they live so they can have fertility coverage. RESOLVE explains coverage of the 15 states.[14]

In addition, a bill to create a tax credit for the out-of-pocket costs associated with infertility treatment has been recently introduced in the United States Senate (2011).[15] This will potentially help thousands of people seeking infertility treatment that otherwise would be out of reach due to inordinate expenses. The bill was brainstormed by RESOLVE, which is best known for their work on expanding insurance coverage for fertility treatment through advocating for state mandates. With the hopes of The Family Act of 2011 bill being passed, if your state currently does not have coverage, you should contact your local representatives and ask them to introduce legislation to require infertility treatment coverage.

Billing

In any case, ask your center of choice how they handle their billing. Our center was fortunate to have a dedicated person that looked up every patient's insurance and called their company to find out their benefits. She would go over all aspect of their coverage with patients and have them sign an explanation of their benefits. And if, due to limited insurance coverage, if you were a self-paying patient, you would know ahead of time what payment is needed up front before beginning treatment. Unfortunately, not all centers have a dedicated person to do this work. So it is up to the patient to find out their coverage. The nurses at times may need to call your insurance for certain parts of treatment. But, given the wide ranges of insurance plans available and the diversity of the patients, it is impossible to expect the nurses to know all the important details.

Some fertility clinics have payment plans; others offer risk sharing or money-back guarantees if infertility treatment is unsuccessful (IVF procedures) (though you have to qualify for this type of program). Be sure you check everything out before signing on the dotted line. Infertility, especially IVF, is very expensive.

Labs

You should ask the specialist about their laboratories. Fertility clinics should have both an Andrology lab and an Embryology lab; the former does semen analysis and sperm washing for Artificial Insemination and the latter handles the care and transfer of embryos during IVF. These labs should be certified by the state as well as by a national organization like the College of American Pathologists (CAP) and Joint Commission and the American Society for Reproductive Medicine (ASRM). Certified labs reflect a good quality control program and that they run a tight ship.

Keep Your Options Open

Some couples start at one center and find they are not happy with their choice. You can always leave and find another. We had a fair amount of patients that came to us from other centers for a number of reasons. This isn't necessarily a reflection on a given center. But, as I mentioned, each couple's situation is unique and they must find the program that suits their unique needs. One couple expressed how the first center they tried had made them feel like they were just a number. The male partner said the specialist indicated that until the female partner had a gastric bypass (because she was overweight), adding to the fact that this male partner had a low sperm count, there was nothing they could do. They left that center devastated. They desperately wanted a child! But they didn't give up. They found another center in which the specialist felt differently and said they could help. Make sure you are happy with your choice, if not move on to another.

Chapter 3
Do I Need Infertility Counseling?

The following introductory section captures a blog post published in *Psychology Today* by Connie Shapiro. I include it here with only minor alterations for readability:[16]

> *Since the recent publication of my book* When You're Not Expecting,[17] *many people have approached me to ask about the counseling experience: How to know when counseling is a good "next step"? How do I access a counselor experienced with infertility issues? What costs may be involved? What should I expect romp the counseling experience? The common thread that is present in these conversations is the fundamental question: "Since I feel like I'm going crazy, is counseling likely to be of any help?"*
>
> These are very important questions. Since I have provided counseling to hundreds of couples and individuals grappling with infertility, I know all too well the kinds of barriers that can prevent people from seeking help for the emo-

tional fallout of infertility. You'll hear throughout the book that infertility is stressful. It is my job to inform and prepare you as much as possible so that once you begin the process you'll be well positioned to know what to expect. Most infertility centers have professional counseling, psychologists and support groups. It is important to be proactive as a couple to learn as much as you can and when confusion arises or you face bumps along the way, you will know there is help out there. Today we'll begin with how to get started in this process.

Getting Started

This is an experience for which you probably have had no preparation. This also is an experience for which you lack a road map, so looming out there in the future is the fear of the unknown and whether you'll have the emotional strength to emerge from the infertility journey unscathed. I think readers would agree with me that the infertility experience is filled with stress. Researchers say the emotional pain a person goes through with infertility is similar to someone having cancer. Who to tell, how much to tell, how to cope with the fertile world, how to communicate with loved ones and health care providers, how to juggle treatment and personal life and, above all, how to bear the interminable waiting: all of this presses in on the couple who faces infertility. The list could be yet more extensive. The point is, it doesn't take long before infertility becomes a ruling force in your life. Anyone who has been infertile for any period of time will be quick to say the experience changes you. The question you will want to ask yourself is: at what point in this process do you want to seek out a counselor to help you cope more effectively with the inevitable stresses? Knowing that infertility will change you, do you want a counselor by your side to help you find new ways to handle the present and to think about the future? And do you see counseling as something for yourself, or is your partner also interested in being involved? You may want to seek a counselor when you are thinking about it all day long and infertility is taking over your life.

Infertility can hurt your relationship; it can be a drain to both of you. This is the time when you need one another and support each other. I heard many times from my patients "Oh, he (or she) is the one who is infertile, not me." I have said this more than once: this is not the time to blame one another. Communication is important and it is imperative that you keep these lines open. Women tend to show more outward emotions and may prefer to talk things through. Men, on the other hand, tend to want to be problem solvers and may not feel the same empathy when there is a failed cycle.

Since I happen to believe in keeping a finger on one's emotional pulse, I would first encourage you to discuss with your partner how each of you feels you are handling the stresses of your infertility. What are the primary stressors for each of you? What do you find difficult to discuss with one another? What are your worst fears about the way infertility will affect you? What sources of support do you have? Many other questions will inevitably arise in your conversations once you begin to open up and face this process. If you find yourself talking openly and honestly with some degree of hopefulness, then you can give yourselves high marks for empathy and self-awareness. If, however, you determine that some issues are causing you emotional pain that needs attention, there are several options to consider.

Communication, Local Support, Infertility Counseling

First, continue to keep open communication with your partner about these topics. So what if your conversation with your loved one is filled with fears, misgivings, tears or apprehensions on at least some of the topics you are discussing? This would suggest to me that at least one of you is hurting, at least one of you feels inadequate or confused about how to soothe your partner, and at least one of you is feeling emotionally overwhelmed on some level. Whether this means that you rarely discuss these issues with one another (usually for fear that the tears will turn to torrents), or that you are often reaching out for comfort that cannot be met by your partner alone, these are signals that you need more emotional support than you are getting.

Second, join a local infertility support group. RESOLVE's web site[18] lists support groups by regions in the U.S., and the Infertility Awareness Association of Canada (IAAC) http://www.iaac.ca does the same for support groups in Canada. In addition, many communities sponsor their own peer-led support groups and beyond that, many infertility clinics offer support groups for their patients.

A third option is to make a preliminary appointment with an infertility counselor. This will give you an opportunity to check out your comfort level with this individual and ascertain whether this is someone with whom you can communicate your struggles and difficulties when they arise. The initial appointment will also give the counselor an opportunity to see you and your partner at a time when you are managing well, which will give him or her a point of reference during future sessions during rough patches. A preliminary appointment will give all parties the opportunity to discuss the future availability of the counselor, as well as practices that you need to know: fees, insurance coverage, length of sessions (usually 50 minutes), and whether the counselor has a preference for working with individuals or couples. If after this initial visit you do not feel sufficiently comfortable with this counselor as the one with whom you would like to work in the future, then continue your quest until you find someone in whom you have more confidence. Waiting for a crisis is no way to pursue this quest.

Counselors are accustomed to clients who are tearful on their first visit, who say "I think I'm going crazy!" by way of introduction, and who are searching for coping skills that elude them in the journey of their infertility. So if this description fits you, your options include inquiring about whether your infertility clinic or physician's practice can provide or refer you to infertility counseling services. If they don't, then you will need to do independent detective work in your community to locate a counselor. Resources to help with this may include the medical social worker at an area hospital, your religious leader, any infertile friends in whom you have confided, as well as listings that may appear on the websites of RESOLVE or IAAC. Even contacting a number listed under "mental health services" in the yellow pages or "googling" infertility counselors with the name of your town may yield a contact number that could give answers to your questions about whether there are experienced infertility counselors in your community. This will take time and requires patience. But it is well worth the effort if it enables you to connect with someone who can help you with these emotional burdens.

Some individuals or couples are so consumed with sadness and depression that it may take emergency intervention to jolt them into getting help and recognizing the depth of their pain. Under these circumstances, when the inability to function or suicidal gestures becomes evident, the resolve to find help must be more immediate. An initial evaluation by a psychiatrist is an important first step, with the likelihood of prompt follow-up by a mental health professional. The initial contact may be through a telephone call to your local mental health clinic where you must firmly request an immediate appointment (that very day). If you are incapable of doing this, it is important to render permission for a loved one to do this on your behalf and with your permission. If scheduling an immediate appointment is not successful, you can make a trip to the emergency room of your hospital where a psychiatric evaluation should be made available. It is far more important to get immediate services in a crisis, and ultimately to learn about the counseling resources in your community once the initial crisis has been addressed.

Briefly, below I have listed different kinds of counselors you may want to pursue (some will refer to themselves as therapists), including their titles and their training:

Psychiatrists: medical doctors who can offer mental health diagnoses and can write prescriptions for anxiety, depression and other conditions. It is important to inquire of the psychiatrist, and of your pharmacist, about the effects of any prescribed medication may have on a developing fetus. Some psychiatrists offer counseling, but it is more likely that a psychiatrist will refer you to one of the professionals listed below.

Psychologists: these professionals possess master's degrees and often Ph.D.s in counseling and mental health related fields, but cannot prescribe medication. They have counseling expertise gained through their education, internships and post-degree supervised clinical experience.

Social workers: these professionals also possess master's degrees, having acquired counseling expertise through clinical supervision during internships and possibly post-degree experience. Social workers often have skills in individual and family counseling, promoting couple communication, addressing issues of loss, advocacy and helping clients to find appropriate community resources.

Marriage and family therapists: these professions also possess master's degrees, having acquired their counseling expertise through clinical supervision during internships and possibly post-degree experience. They provide individual counseling, couple counseling and family counseling.

It is possible that any of the counselors listed above, who are licensed in their states of residence, may be eligible to receive insurance reimbursement for providing services to you. This differs in each location, and a call to your insurance provider should be able to determine whether the counselor is considered a provider in that particular system. If money presents a barrier, there are other options you can pursue. You can ask a counselor whether s/he can offer you a sliding fee scale (flexible fees depending on an individual's financial circumstances). If individual counselors in your area cannot offer this flexibility, sometimes agency counselors (at Family and Children's Services and Mental Health Agencies) offer a sliding fee scale. Should none of these options be available, I would suggest a very open conversation with your counselor about an initial partial payment plan, with a repayment plan built in. Another option might be to see the counselor less frequently than weekly, thereby incurring less cost.

I know for any readers who looked at my "getting started" title and expected to whiz through this portion, might be feeling overwhelmed at the scope and complexity of this process. But remember, what I have tried to do is to depict the process in sufficient detail so that you can picture your own circumstances in the options presented. In truth, you don't need to digest everything in this section. Simply appropriate those parts that apply to you.

And, while you're digesting, I'll mention that my book (*When You're Not Expecting*) offers therapeutic tips at the end of every chapter. So while you are considering whether to and when to seek a counselor, you may find that the book acquaints you with the process of learning effective coping and communication skills over the course of the infertility journey."[19]

Extenuating Circumstances

A third party: It's very possible that the clinic you choose will have on staff an infertility counselor(s), which would eliminate much in the way of added stress and complications. In fact, your RE will recommend or may require that you see a counselor before certain treatments. For example, if a couple is going to use egg or sperm donors, they will need counseling. People who want to be egg donors and sperm donors are required to undergo a mental health overview before they will be considered for donation. Using a donor or surrogate brings into play many issues that one might not necessarily think about when the process begins. It is imperative that you, as a couple, feel comfortable before receiving a donation or—in the case of the donor—before giving over this intimate part of your life. This is when a third person enters your infertility corner, which can share the struggle, but which also can complicate the already-complex emotions. There are enough feelings of loss using you own gametes[20] when starting an IVF cycle. These only become more acute when you use the egg or the sperm of a third party, or when that third party is carrying your child. You want to be well apprised of such complexities before embarking on this level of intervention in your infertility journey. You both need to feel good about this decision. A counselor will serve to highlight points that you haven't thought about.

There are other situations in which people's lifestyles may differ, creating unforeseeable complications in their desire to have children. The RE will have cases such as these consult an infertility counselor before any treatment is given.

A polyamorous relationship

A recent episode of the television drama *Private Practice* highlights a far-fetched but altogether plausible complexity can arise among loved ones who want to have a child. In this case, the situation involved three people: two females and a gentleman. All three had gone to consult with their RE in the effort to lay out their plan for having a family together. The three had it all figured out: one female would donate the eggs; one would be the surrogate; and the male would give his sperm. The three of them wanted to be a part of this baby's creation and life.

They had the appointment with the therapist and it came to light that the male was not simply a "directed donor."[21] The three of them were sharing what is called a "polyamory relationship"– the practice, desire, or acceptance of having more than one intimate relationship at a time with the knowledge and consent of everyone involved.[22] Polyamorous arrangements are varied, reflecting choices and philosophies of the individuals who compose them. The distinguishing feature of polyamory from traditional forms of non-monogamy (i.e. infidelity) is the ideology that openness, goodwill, truthful communication, and ethical behavior prevail among all the parties involved.[23]

In this instance (referring again to the television program) the two females were examined and both had ultrasounds. It was discovered that one of them had contracted genital tuberculosis, which, evidently, she had picked up on a recent trip to South America. The ultrasound revealed that she was infertile and would not be able to donate her eggs or carry the baby because of the damage caused by the disease. The fallopian tubes, which transport eggs from the ovaries to the uterus, are the most common organs involved in genital tuberculosis, which blocks the passages and leads to permanent infertility. This woman was devastated, understandably.[24]

As the story unfolds the infertile female now insisted she did not want to have a child according to the original plan as the three had originally conceived it. Instead, she wanted to adopt. Though this scenario sounds like (and is) a made-for-TV script, the story is plausible and could very well happen.

In another case, a woman who was undergoing IVF —in addition to using her own eggs for herself—donated her eggs to her infertile sister. Both underwent IVF during the same cycle, using their respective husbands' sperm. In this case, the donating sister did not get pregnant, and her infertile sister receiving also did not get pregnant, but just think if she did: How would her sister giving the eggs feel? It seems appropriate to highlight that all parties in this scenario required extra help in the way of therapy.

As long as I have been in this field, I have seen cases like these and many others that warranted solid, intense and honest consultation with a therapist. There is more to think about than you can imagine once this process begins. So when the RE wants you to see a therapist, be assured that there is a reason for it. You'll discover things that you may have not thought about and in the end will be grateful.

/

t May Not Happen

This may sound harsh but I need to discuss the possibility that, after all the counseling and related procedures, you still may not get pregnant. We in the infertility field want everyone who undertakes this journey to be successful. And most couples are. Yet, there is a small percentage that aren't as fortunate. What if you don't get pregnant and you make the decision of a childless life? You've gone through years of infertility treatment and you don't want to adopt. A counselor can help you process your emotions. I myself did some IUI treatments but didn't want to go on further with IVF. We as a couple felt that we did try something and now could close that door.

Only you and your partner can ultimately decide: "When do I stop treatment?" It's your decision! So take it slow and listen to your heart and your partner's heart. As you read *Sperm Tales*, keep in mind there are no guarantees about getting pregnant. Your RE will do as much as he/she can to help you. This book, I hope, will introduce you to the various ups and downs of treatment so that you can be well educated on the subject and be aware of various avenues for any emotional and psychological help you may need.

Chapter 4
Alternative Treatments for De-Stressing and Coping

As mentioned, infertility can fundamentally change you and your partner's lives. So knowing this ahead of time, patients should be constantly aware of their feelings and continue to communicate with each other and your specialist. If the standard options for addressing the toll this takes, as enumerated in the previous chapter, do not work for you or are otherwise inaccessible, several alternative forms of treatment exist that can relieve stress throughout this roller–coaster process: acupuncture, yoga, and Reiki.[25]

Acupuncture

The following section on acupuncture was written by the Acupuncturist at our center named Zhenzhen Zhang.[26]

Acupuncture for Infertility
"Last week, a 39-year old woman walked into my office and asked me if acupuncture could help her to get pregnant. As with all my patients, I spend

some time asking detailed information about her, including her menstrual history and general health condition. She has always had irregular and painful menstrual cycles. I also learned that she has failed five IVF cycles in the past, and her doctor would not able to begin another cycle because her Follicle Stimulating Hormone (FSH) levels are too high. I proposed she begin a treatment plan as early as she could for three months, for acupuncture treatments once per week, except the second week of her menstrual cycle, with two treatments. I also answered many of her questions, which are commonly asked by my patients:

How does acupuncture treat infertility?

Acupuncture has been utilized for thousands of years to help woman become pregnant. To explain with Chinese Medicine theory, acupuncture frees the blockage of energy flow, warms cold energy, and removes the stasis that causes infertility; the acupuncture needles can be placed on the head, abdomen and extremities, stimulating signals that acting on nerves and the endocrine system to make desired physiological changes. These explanations fit into the fundamental theories of Chinese Medicine, but are difficult to understand in the context of Western medical beliefs. However, in recent years, more and more research has been done to discover the underlying mechanisms of Chinese Medicine through Western medical methods.

Recent research results: Acupuncture can reduce stress, anxiety and even depression: for women with unknown causes of infertility, stress maybe the biggest contributing factor. Every infertility patient experiences a certain amount of stress, which can negatively effect on the ovulatory menstrual cycle, because increased stress hormones can interfere with the reproductive hormone system. In my clinic, it is very common for irregular menstrual cycles to become regular after acupuncture treatment. Reducing stress is the basic strategy for the infertility treatment protocol.

Acupuncture can also rebalance hormones. As we know, infertility can be caused by irregularity in hormones, such as estradiol (E2), follicle-stimulating hormone (FSH), progesterone, or luteinizing hormone (LH), either it too high or too low. Hormonal irregularity can then cause ovarian and or uterine malfunction. Thus, acupuncture regulates the hypothalamic-pituitary-ovarian axis, the source of women's ovulatory and fertility hormones.

Lastly, acupuncture has been shown to increase blood flow in reproductive organs to improve their functions. In the April 2002 issue of *Fertility and Sterility*, two studies in Germany and China reported that adding acupuncture to IVF treatments can improve the women's chances of becoming pregnant. Many subsequent researches have confirmed this.

How often acupuncture treatment is needed?

The menstrual cycle is divided into four phases for most women: menstruation, pre-ovulation, ovulation and luteal phases. Usually, patients need treatment one or two times per week, and more treatments can generally be more beneficial. For patients unable to come in twice per week, I suggest her to come twice during the pre-ovulation phase. Each session of treatment method and selection of acupuncture points used will be different according to the phase of the cycle and the patient's specific condition.

Do I need Chinese herbal medicine in addition to acupuncture treatments?

I may recommend Chinese herbal medicine in combination with acupuncture for those not taking Western medicine. This is particularly recommended for patients who are only able to come once per week for acupuncture treatment. Patients can consult with their primary care physician in deciding whether to take herbs or not. For patients undergoing modern fertility procedure such as IVF or IUI, herbs are not recommended, in order to prevent any interacting effects.

What other treatments methods are used?

Beside acupuncture needles, we also may use electro-acupuncture, ear acupuncture, the heating method (infrared lamp or moxa), etc. The type of recommended treatment depends on the phase of menstrual cycle and the patient's condition.

When should I start acupuncture treatment?

We know acupuncture has both short term and long-term effects on the body. The short-term effects are usually apparent in stress-related psychological issues and pain. The long-term effects require frequent treatments and many sessions; the accumulated short-term effects become long-term effects. Many people have experienced improvements in pain or mood swings immediately after treatment, but the effects only last for a few days and the conditions return to their original state before the subsequent acupuncture session a week later. However, after more frequent sessions of acupuncture treatment, the condition becomes more stable with long lasting results.

For complicated or serious infertility conditions, my suggestion is to begin acupuncture as earlier as possible, in order to maximize both psychological and physical benefits. For patients seeking treatments only during their IUI or IVF cycles, acupuncture can provide positive short-term effects on their cycles.

When should I stop acupuncture treatments?

For most infertility cases, acupuncture can be stopped two weeks after confirmed conception. However, I would suggest continuing acupuncture treatment into the first trimester for patients the following cases: history of miscarriages, signs of early miscarriage, severe morning sickness, and severe emotion swings. Furthermore, treatments can be resumed at any time during pregnancy if other severe psychological or physical issues occur. I specify severe cases, because women undergoing normal pregnancies often have minor and tolerable symptoms, which require no extra care.

Is acupuncture safe, and for what conditions should I seek acupuncture treatment during pregnancy?
  Well-trained acupuncturists are knowledgeable about treating pregnant patients, knowing on which parts of body needles can and cannot be placed and helping patients without causing harm to the pregnancy.
  Common conditions during pregnancy for that acupuncture help include: morning sickness (which does not necessarily occur in the morning), neck tension or pain, headaches, dizziness, lower back pain, sciatica pain, legs edema, emotional and psychiatric issues, sickness, fatigue, overdue pregnancy, breech baby, and some preexisting conditions."

Yoga
  I recently took yoga classes and came to find out my instructor had been an infertility patient at our center. I asked her to write a short portion in this book about how yoga helped her navigate this challenge. Her name is

Paula Wilson and I love her story:

> Yoga brings together physical and mental disciplines to achieve peacefulness of body and mind, helping you relax and manage stress and anxiety. Through yoga techniques, you are able to redirect your attention to focus on yourself, your movement and your breathing. All of these elements combine to help relieve stress, and help to realign and balance out your body's systems. "These are some of the reasons why many infertile couples have found yoga to be helpful for them. Each yoga exercise focuses on a different area of your body and works in conjunction with your mind and your breath."[27]
>
> "Studies report that women who practice yoga are twice as likely to get pregnant because yoga decreases stress and increases blood circulation to the reproductive organs. Among American women, 7.3 million suffer from infertility. And though many options exist that can help couples conceive, their long paths to parenthood can be painful."[28]
>
> Infertility can be overwhelming, depressing, demanding, frustrating and extremely stressful.[29] Unfortunately, I felt all of these emotions in the almost five years it took to conceive my son by going through the infertility process. Those five years felt like an eternity. I felt so alone, even though my husband was very supportive. I felt like I was the only one who couldn't conceive a child. Almost all of my friends had children already, and yet we

were still trying. My biological clock was ticking. I had a stressful job at the time and was completely miserable. I persevered because I wanted to have a child so desperately. So, I subjected myself to all of the tests and interventions, until finally, one day, a few weeks after IVF, I got the call that I had dreamed about for years. I was finally pregnant at 37! My life changed from that day on. I had already left my job a few months prior and had made the decision to become a yoga instructor. I had practiced yoga for many years and always loved it. So I felt it was a perfect time to learn more about it and be able to teach and help others with their yoga practice. Also, being pregnant, I wanted to experience all of the benefits of yoga for myself and my unborn child.[30]

The yoga training was a wonderful experience. I learned a tremendous amount about yoga and how beneficial it is for everyone. I learned how to breathe properly and how to relax and relieve stress, while strengthening my muscles, increasing my flexibility and balance. It was great to be pregnant during the training, as I was able to learn about the importance of yoga with regard to the mind-body relationship through exercise and relaxation during pregnancy. I became so much more flexible, calm and focused during my pregnancy.

I had a beautiful baby boy in December 2004. We thought he would be our only child as it was so difficult to conceive him. We agreed that we didn't want to go through the stress of infertility treatments again. Miraculously, a year and a half later, I found out I was pregnant again without any medical intervention! We had a beautiful daughter two years and two months later. I was a few months shy of turning forty.

I was practicing yoga as much as I could after my son was born and started teaching yoga at the end of my pregnancy. Unfortunately, I broke my foot in my last trimester. I was unable to teach for several months, which was extremely difficult for me. Once I was back on my feet and able to practice again, I began teaching again. Although I wasn't practicing as much as I was during my teacher training, I was still doing yoga at least a few times a week.

I honestly feel that my yoga practice allowed my body to have an easier delivery, by helping me with breathing and improving my flexibility. Yoga also helped me reduce my anxiety, helped me to relax and got my body ready for pregnancy again. I don't think we would have had another child if I hadn't been devoted to yoga. I am so thankful that I found yoga and for all that it has done for me over the past ten years. I was able to practice and teach yoga through my entire second pregnancy up until about a week before I delivered my daughter. I only took a few weeks off and got back to teaching as soon as I was able.

Several years later, I am still teaching five-to-six yoga classes per week and I have expanded my classes to make yoga available for everyone. I now teach several children's yoga classes as well as adult classes for all levels.

Yoga has truly changed my life and has made such a positive impact on it. It has made me a better person overall. I am thankful for my two beautiful children and consider them both miracle babies."[31]

Paschimottanasana

A particularly helpful exercise, known as Paschimottanasana or the "Seated Forward Bend," relieves stress and mild depression; stimulates the liver, kidneys, ovaries and uterus; improves digestion; and helps to relieve symptoms of menstrual discomfort and menopause. Further, it soothes headaches and settles anxiety.

Sit on the floor and you bend forward and reach your toes. The pose stretches the spine, shoulders and hamstrings.

Reiki[32]

Another natural fertility treatment that is on the rise in popularity is Reiki therapy. Reiki treatments are based on the channeling of positive energy so as to promote overall health. (Defined in more detail below.) As such, Reiki healing is a natural fertility method that can help improve your chances of getting pregnant by minimizing health problems and conditions that can hinder your fertility.

What is Reiki Therapy?

Reiki treatment is a natural therapy that is used to improve overall well being and to promote healing in the body. Reiki therapy is an ancient Japanese healing method whose primary objective is to balance the energy (*chi*) in the body. Reiki seeks to encourage energy flow so as to foster self-healing.

During a Reiki treatment session a practitioner uses gentle hand movements, hovering his or her hands just above the patient's body, including the head, shoulders, stomach, back, legs and feet. According to the principles of Reiki, these movements channel positive energy from the hands of the practitioner to that of the patient. These hand movements are often performed without any bodily contact from the therapist, whose energy, proponents say, can actually be felt coming from their hands.

One of the greatest healing health benefits of Reiki is stress reduction and relaxation. As noted above, stress reduction triggers our body's natural healing process and improves health and the well being of the entire physical, emotional and psychic/spiritual body. The result it is a holistic, natural (and non-invasive) system of promoting wholeness of mind, body and spirit.

Reiki Therapy and Infertility

Because Reiki therapy works to improve overall physical and mental health, including reproductive health, it can likewise improve your chances of getting pregnant. As such, Reiki therapy can help to improve your health so as to minimize conditions and illnesses that can contribute to infertility. For example, Reiki therapy can help to maintain good reproductive health that is beneficial for both men and women. Your therapist can show you how you and your partner can do this together to help you as a couple going through infertility. Also, because stress is often linked to fertility problems, Reiki therapy can benefit those for whom stress is contributing factor to problems getting pregnant. By promoting good preconception health, Reiki treatment can also help to foster good prenatal health.

Reiki Therapy Session

An average Reiki treatment lasts from between 60 minutes to 90 minutes. In order to be effective, it is recommended that you start with one or two sessions per week. Ensure that your Reiki therapy practitioner is qualified, by inquiring about his/her qualifications, including where he/she was trained. You should also ask to see qualification certificates and diplomas.

I myself benefited from Reiki treatments when I had to get an MRI despite acute claustrophobia. The treatments relaxed me and helped me through the one hour MRI test. Some of our patients had the Reiki therapist come to the clinic to give her a treatment before the woman had her IUI.

In sum, please explore these or some other means of relaxation treatment when you are in an infertility program. Life is stressful enough. I know these will help you during your treatments.

Chapter 5
What to Expect – What is ART?

Some fertility programs are located in a large hospital setting and some in a more intimate clinic setting. The staff can consist of four to five Reproductive Endocrinologists (RE), Urologists, Nurses, Embryologists and professional counselors. Larger programs could have a larger staff.

The clinic will have a laboratory, which may be called an Andrology Lab; Andrology is the study of the male reproductive organs. The lab consists of three to five medical technologists, depending upon the size of the clinic and whether or not it specializes in Andrology. The Andrology lab performs the blood tests and measures hormones; it performs semen analysis and sperm washing for IUI, and may possibly have a sperm bank. The clinic may have an IVF lab or be affiliated with a hospital that has the lab. An IVF lab consists of many embryologists, which perform the intricate testing that goes along with IVF.

The Pivotal Role of Your Nurse

Depending on the program, a nurse is assigned to one or two specialists. The RE works together with you as a couple, and will order blood work and other diagnostic tests. But when it comes to physical exams the RE examines only the female partner. If the male has an abnormal semen analysis or any conditions that relate to the male reproductive system, he'll be sent to an Urologist for an examination.

The nurse that is assigned to a couple in a fertility program remains involved with the patients at every step, building communication and trusting relationships with the patients. Sandy Vance, nurse manager at Women's Health Center has said, "Infertility has been compared to a terminal illness and when a woman has tried everything and cannot get pregnant, she begins to experience grief, shock, denial, isolation, depression and guilt. We work to get the woman to a place where she can understand what her status is." (This is perhaps the only field in which nurses work more with the patients than the physicians.) Once you have the first consult with the specialist, the nurse then becomes the person with whom you will communicate the most on a monthly, weekly or even daily basis. The nurse that you'll be assigned to will give you a packet containing information on testing. It may also contain orders for your testing, instructions on giving injections, operational hours of the center, and who to call in an emergency. Please read this information and keep it in a safe spot at home.

These nurses are on their phones most of the day, answering questions, encouraging, or giving instructions to their patients. One of the hardest calls they make to a patient is that her pregnancy test came out negative and it doesn't get any easier. The best call is the one that delivers the news to the patient that her pregnancy is positive. Nurses are so excited and make that call first.

In either case, as one of our nurses at our Women's Health Center, Paula Ayers, has said, "The most gratifying compliment I can receive is when a woman does not achieve success in conceiving, despite all of our efforts, and she thanks us for the respect and supportive approach to her care."

One patient, who went through the program at the age of 40 and was diagnosed with old eggs, was able to get pregnant after her first IVF cycle. She said, "It may sound easy but until you are the one going through it you can't appreciate the kindness of the nurses. Even on my lowest day, thinking this wasn't going to happen, Sandy found something positive we could hold on to."[33]

As you can see, nurses in a fertility program grow very attached to their patients and work very hard, with great compassion, to help patients navigate the ongoing ups-and-downs of an infertility program.

I posed this question on Facebook to some fertility nurses: *In a perfect world, what would make your day-to-day job easier when it comes to caring for your patients?*

Sandy Vance (mentioned above) responded: "We all like it when patients ask questions, because it shows that they really want to understand their treatment. But it would be helpful if they would read all of the materials we send home with them. They really are helpful in explaining the process."

How the Process Begins

Sperm Tales is going to take you through what is involved in the Infertility program. Whether it involves choosing a center; what to expect in the initial consult and diagnostic testing (for both partners); to finding out where you are with your fertility and making a plan with the specialist that you both feel comfortable with; this book will guide you through each phase.

The first phase will start you with one of the following Assisted Reproductive Technologies (ART) procedures and may progress to others depending on your success. These procedures include and not limited to Intrauterine Insemination (IUI) and In Vitro Fertilization (IVF), also known as the "Test Tube Baby." Beyond that, IVF can break down to include other techniques (such as, for example Intracytoplasmic Sperm Injection, ICSI). Below are a few brief descriptions of both IUI and IVF (to go into more detail later).

What happens in an IUI?

The Intrauterine Insemination (IUI) procedure is a simple procedure that takes little time and involves minimum discomfort. At the time of ovulation the sperm is collected and processed. The sperm is then placed in a catheter and is placed in the female's uterus. It is very important that this procedure, also known as artificial insemination, occurs with ovulation. Using the over-the-counter ovulation kits can easily monitor the time of ovulation. The hormone Luteinizing Hormone (LH) is measured, noting when it spikes. This indicates ovulation has occurred and the female is at her most fertile time. The IUIs are performed seven days a week and take only about one hour. The males collect the specimens in the morning and drop it off at the lab. (Some centers prefer the males to collect the specimen at the center.) The lab performs a sperm wash to the specimen, wherein the non-motile sperm is separated from the motile sperm and other debris from the semen. The female partner returns to the center around 11:30 a.m. to 12:00 noon for IUI procedure. The washed specimen is placed in a catheter and is inserted through the cervix into the uterus where the specimen is released. The procedure is very similar to getting a pap smear. The patient relaxes in the exam room for about 10 to 15 minutes after the procedure and then she can resume her daily routine. The nurse instructs her to notify the nurse in two weeks if she has not gotten her menstrual cycle. At that time her blood will be drawn for a pregnancy test.

Medications to Help Ovulation

Ovulation remains one of the most common female infertility disorders. Thus, ovulation induction is a common infertility treatment using fertility medications to help stimulate the ovaries and cause ovulation. This can help many women increase the chance of conceiving. Two of the common medications used are Clomid and FSH injectable medications.

Clomid

Clomid is the most common fertility drug used to stimulate the ovarian function. It is an oral medication with a chemical structure very close to estrogen. It works by triggering the body to produce the follicle-stimulating hormone (FSH), which is responsible for the developing ovarian follicles and maturing the eggs inside those follicles. Clomid is taken for five days. During that time the patient may be instructed to have an ultrasound to monitor the ovaries. To maximize the chances for conception, when ovulation occurs, the sperm must be present either during intercourse or by an IUI within 24 to 38 hours.

Gonadotropin (FSH) Medications

Gonadotropin injections are another option, which have significant advantages, as well as some disadvantages, to using Clomid. (There are many good FSH medications on the market and your RE will decide which one to take.) FSH injections are more potent than Clomid and will produce more follicles. When doing IUIs it is optimal if the patient produces two to three follicles because the potential exists for each follicle to become an embryo. Blood work and ultrasound monitoring help the RE determine how the patient's body receives the FSH medications. Advantages of FSH medications over Clomid include the increase in estrogen, which increases the cervical mucus. This helps to nourish the sperm and enables them to swim to the eggs. The increase in estrogen helps increase the lining of the uterus for implantation.

However the disadvantage of FSH medication over Clomid include more visits to the center for blood and ultrasound monitoring. The average woman takes the injections for seven days. This means making about five visits to the center for blood tests and ultrasounds. The blood measures the amount of estrogen, which will increase because of the FSH medication. The ultrasound enables the medical team to view the number of follicles present as well as how large they are. FSH medications are much more expensive than the price of Clomid.[34] There is also a higher risk of having multiple births with FSH medication over Clomid. For example those who take FSH medications will see 20 percent increased chance of having twins, as compared to six to eight percent for those who use Clomid.[35] Patients who take FSH medication also have an increased risk of ovarian hyperstimulation (OHSS), when the ovaries become swollen and painful. There are mild to severe cases of ovarian hyperstimulation. If this occurs you'll be watched closely by your RE.

What happens in IVF?

IVF is more involved than an IUI. An IUI is less invasive and the cost is much less. This procedure differs from an IUI because the eggs are removed from the female's body. The female will take the gonadotropins FSH injections that will stimulate the ovaries to produce as many eggs as possible. The eggs will be removed surgically, which is called the retrieval, and then placed in a petri dish where your partner's sperm will be washed and placed with your eggs. The dish is incubated and evaluated a few days later to see how many eggs fertilized. The female returns for an embryo transfer, which is where a certain number of embryos will be placed back or transferred into the uterus. The embryos will be placed in a catheter like the sperm for the IUI and placed in the uterus. You'll return to the center in approximately 14 days after the procedure for a pregnancy blood test. The success rate for IVF is higher than IUI.

Which procedure you start with depends on the results of your initial testing (for both of you), insurance coverage, and how aggressive you want to be, depending upon your, or lack of success at other clinics. This will all be discussed with your specialist.

Infertility has its own vernacular, or terminology. *Sperm Tales* has included a helpful glossary at the end of the book, which you can refer to at any time you may get confused.

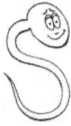

panky says:

"The wife says to her partner:
'You get a lounge and
I get a speculum and a catheter!'"

Chapter 6
Preconception Care

We have taken a cursory look at how to be prepared for the medical procedures related to infertility treatment. In this chapter I want to examine what you can be doing as a patient to help your body prepare for this process.

I've been asked by a number of patients, "What can I do on my end to help my body prepare?" This side of the equation is as important as the medical side. We know that a healthy diet and lifestyle are beneficial for all systems of the body. If you and your partner are serious in starting a family, adapting your lifestyles as soon as possible, to reach this goal, is an important first step that will help with your results. Studies have shown a direct correlation between good nutrition and improved quality of sperm.

The following information[36] is taken from an infertility web site, and discusses preparing your body for pregnancy and includes advice on nutrition, screening and change in lifestyle. (Bibligraphical citations are retained within the text to reflect it as it appeared in the original article.)

Improving your chances by preparing for pregnancy

It is important that you and your partner get off to the best possible start for the much-wanted pregnancy. There are important links between preconception health and positive IVF outcomes. Preparing for pregnancy will not only increase your chance of achieving a pregnancy but may also decrease the risk of complications to both mother and fetus. Researchers from the University Medical Center in The Netherlands reported that 96 percent of women who attended a preconception clinic before undergoing IVF had three or more lifestyle problems and risk factors such as obesity, smoking, recreation drugs and alcohol (*Journal of Advanced Nursing*, 2012). Increasing numbers of women with often complex medical conditions such as women who had renal transplant or cardiac surgery are now becoming pregnant or seeking fertility treatment, these women should receive pre-pregnancy counseling, ideally by multidisciplinary team involving their specialists and obstetric physicians.

What lifestyle changes should you consider when you plan for a pregnancy?

Weight and nutrition

It is essential to eat a balanced healthy diet with fresh fruits, green vegetables and plenty of water. Avoid eating processed food, as it contains flavoring and additives. Diet rich in Omega-3s can significantly decrease natural killer cell activity and suppress the production of Tumor Necrosis Factor (TNF) alpha cytokines (Frank et al 2001; Gazvani et al 2001). Being overweight or underweight can affect normal ovulation; reduce the chance of getting pregnant, increase pregnancy complications and the risks associated with anesthesia. If your body mass index is above 30 you need a supervised weight loss program involving dietary advice and exercise. Obese women take longer to conceive and are at higher risk of miscarriage than ordinary women. If your body mass index is less than 20 then you may also need to go on a sensible eating program to correct it. Restoration of body weight may help resume ovulation and restore fertility.

Give up smoking.
If this is difficult, cut down as much as possible. Cigarette smoking is harmful to the woman's ovaries (smoking has been linked to premature ovarian aging; Kinney 2007). Women who smoke reduce their chance of successful pregnancy by approximately 40 percent, compared with non-smokers. Smoking reduces implantation and pregnancy rates (Neal et al., 2005,. Human Reproduction). Smoking also adversely affects live birth rates equivalent to increased female age by 10 years (Linsten et al, 2005. Human Reproduction, Salihu et al. Early Hun Dev 2007; Gray et al BMJ 2009). Furthermore, pregnant smokers are more likely to have low birth rate babies and preterm birth etc. It has also been associated with an increased risk of miscarriage, placenta previa (low-lying placenta) and abruption placenta (separation of a normally sited placenta from its attachment into the womb).

Reduce or eliminate consumption of alcohol.

Alcohol consumption may affect ovulation. In addition, there is an increasing body of evidence suggesting harm to the fetus from alcohol consumption during pregnancy including increased rate of miscarriage, growth retardation, prematurity, and developmental delay. Furthermore, excess alcohol during pregnancy is associated with fetal abnormalities such as 'Fetal Alcohol Syndrome'. The syndrome can lead to learning and physical disabilities and behavioral problems.

Do not use recreational drugs: marijuana, cocaine.

The use of cannabis by women in the year before IVF treatment is associated with a reduction of the number of eggs collected (Klonoff-Cohen et al, 2006. American Journal of Obstetrics and Gynecology). It is also associated with preterm birth and low birth weight. Heroin is associated with miscarriage, growth restriction and preterm birth.

Antidepressant medication

Women who are taking antidepressants should consult their OB-GYN and psychiatrist about continuing the medication while trying to conceive and being pregnant. There are pros and cons about this. Severely depressed pregnant women may not take care of themselves properly, not eating well and perhaps not keeping doctor's appointments. They also may tend to drink and smoke while pregnant, which can result in premature births, low birth weights and developmental problems. In an instance such as this, antidepressants may be necessary and some antidepressants are safe. In any case, patients must check with their physicians about this if they are to undergo infertility treatments.

Breast self-examination

This will help to pick up a breast lump. Breast cancer is rare in young women. However, the high levels of hormone estradiol and progesterone produced by the ovarian stimulation drugs could stimulate the growth of a pre-existing cancer. If you find a lump in your breast, your doctor should assess this urgently. He or she will be able to arrange further evaluation and referral to a specialist when necessary.

Stop or reduce the caffeine intake

Caffeine is present in coffee, tea, Coca-Cola, chocolate, etc., and is associated with an increased risk of fetal growth restriction (Care study group 2008 BMJ), miscarriage and low birth rates (Fernandos 1998 and Cnattingius, 2000). Decaffeinated coffee could aggravate the immune system more than caffeinated variety (Mikuls et al. 2003).

Avoid cat litter and under-cooked meat

This reduces the risk of catching toxoplasmosis in pregnancy. Toxoplasmosis may cause brain damage to the fetus.

Keep your mouth as healthy as possible

If you have periodontal disease, get this treated before you become pregnant. There is evidence that treating periodontal disease reduces the risk of having a preterm baby.

Assess your over-all health

If you suffer from a chronic medical condition and are on regular medications such as high blood pressure, epilepsy, diabetes and asthma etc., check with your doctor if these medications are safe in pregnancy. For example, if you are taking Angiotensin Converting Enzyme (ACE) inhibitors, which are high blood pressure drugs such as Ramipril to control high blood pressure, this drug is not safe in pregnancy as it can cause skull abnormalities and renal failure in the fetus. Your doctor may change it to safer drugs such as methyldopa, labetalol or Nifedipine.

Check if you are immune to Rubella (German Measles)

Rubella puts babies at risk of blindness, deafness, mental retardation and heart defect. Women who are susceptible to rubella should be offered rubella vaccination before they become pregnant. Women should avoid conception for a month after Rubella vaccination.

Check if you are immune to chickenpox

Nine out of ten pregnant women (90 percent) in the U.K. are immune to chickenpox. If you are not immune, have the vaccine. The chickenpox vaccination is effective in making nine out of ten women (90 percent) immune.

The vaccination cannot be given during pregnancy and you should avoid getting pregnant for three months after the injection. Primary infection with herpes varicella zoster virus (VZV) in pregnancy may cause maternal mortality or serious complications such as inflammation of the lungs (pneumonia) and inflammation of the brain (encephalitis). It may also cause fetal varicella syndrome, when the chickenpox virus affects the fetus and causes severe birth defects. If you are pregnant and you are not immune, avoid contact with any person who has chickenpox or shingles and to immediately inform healthcare workers of a potential exposure.

Other Precautions

- Check if your cervical smear (PAP test) is in date.
- Check if you have a high blood pressure.
- Check if you are anemic.
- Check if you are diabetic (indicated by sugar in the urine).
- Check if you have got kidney disease (indicated by protein in the urine).
- Check if you have got genital infection (many genital-urinary infection are asymptomatic).
- Test for HIV, Hepatitis B or Hepatitis C, if appropriate, to minimize the viral load[37] and reduce the risk of transmission to the fetus. (These tests are required if doing IVF; patients should check with their nurse.)
- Request certain tests to check for genetic diseases,

especially if there is a history of genetic disorders or for certain ethnicity group, (e.g. Sickle cell, thalassemia and cystic fibrosis. (Most infertility programs are testing now for certain genetic diseases; patients should check with their nurse.)

Occupation

Some occupations may reduce male and female fertility such as bakers, drivers, welders, radiotherapists, agricultural workers and woodworkers. The exposure to heat, X-rays, chemical pesticides, solvents, mercury, phthalates etc. may all contribute to infertility.

Folic acid

It is advisable those women who are contemplating pregnancy should take folic acid (Vitamin B9) in the form of one tablet a day (400 mcg) until the 12th week of pregnancy. This will decrease the risk of neural tube defects such as spina bifida (a hole in the spine) and anencephaly (absent brain) and hydrochephaly (water in the brain). This dose should be increased to 4 mg daily in women who have previously had a baby with a neural tube defect and women who have epilepsy and are taking medication, women who have diabetes and women who have celiac disease.

If you are not very keen to take folic acid tablets you need to eat foods that are rich in folic acid such as spinach, green beans, fortified cornflakes and oranges. Patients should check with their physician.

Advice for men

- Wear loose fitting boxer shorts and trousers.
- Avoid hot baths and take showers instead.
- Cut down smoking and alcohol drinking or stop altogether. Men who smoke heavily or drink too much appear to have lower sperm motility and a higher proportion of abnormal sperm (*Fertility and Sterility*, 2007).
- Maintain a good healthy diet; men consuming omega-3 fatty acids were found to have sperm with a more normal structure and higher concentration (count) than men who consume junk food diets with high levels of saturated fats.
- If overweight they should loose weight.
- Avoid exposure to chemicals and radiations, etc.

Chapter 7
The Initial Consult

You are ready to call the infertility specialist to book the initial consult. You may know of a specialist through a friend or family member. Or, if not, your OB-GYN can recommend an infertility specialist. In the process of looking, always come away with at least a couple of names so you can make the best possible choice. For example, you may feel more comfortable with a female specialist. (Just as a reminder: at this point patients should have notified their insurance company to determine if their plan included infertility coverage.)

If possible it is a very good idea for both partners to meet with the specialist for the first consult. Infertility includes the two of you. It can be a long road and you both can use one another's support. When the two of you enter an infertility program, you'll find that the experience is unlike anything you've ever known before. On the day of your appointment you will be brought into a consult room where you both meet with the specialist. Together you will review the completed paperwork that highlights the female and male's medical history and current medical status. The RE will also need the patient's records sent from the OB-GYN's office; this will be mentioned on the day the patient calls the specialist's office for a consult.

You'll discuss the medical histories and explore the possibilities and options for moving forward. This is the time to ask the specialist any questions you may harbor, whether large or small. You may want to discuss the possibility of multiple births; you will want to ask about that clinic's success rate for IUIs and IVF. (After you've read *Sperm Tales* you will have a good list of preliminary questions for the specialist.)

If this is a second specialist you're seeing in the process of searching for the right one, the RE will want to review some of the preliminary testing you have already undergone. The specialist will ask you questions and outline next steps

The RE may at this time want to do a physical exam to the female. He or she will also start with blood work drawn from the female and discuss scheduling an appointment for a semen analysis on the male partner. These are the beginning tests for any couple (to be discussed).

After the consult you both will be brought down to an exam room were you'll meet the nurse who will be working with you. The nurse will introduce herself and ask if there are any questions (or ask some of her own). She will give an introductory packet and explain what is in it. The packet will contain information that explains all the testing that the patient will need, hours of that clinic's operation, who to call in case of an emergency and other information.

The nurse will explain to the female about some of the testing, which will consist of blood work. Depending on the couple's situation, the male also may have to get blood work. Some of the tests may be scheduled for when the female gets her next menstrual cycle.

Another part of female testing is a Hysteroscopy, which is a test that looks at the uterine lining and Hysterosalpingogram (HSG), which is a test that looks for blockages in the fallopian tubes. The nurse will explain all the details if the female needs these. (The tests will be covered in chapter 9.) The male partner will do a semen analysis unless he had a recent one ordered by the female's OB-GYN.

When the initial testing is complete you'll make a second consult appointment with the specialist to discuss all the results. At this point, together, you will outline and set up a plan for how to move forward.

You may wonder, "How soon can I get started?" It may take a month or two months to get started depending on all your results. Some patients could have cases where they may need some surgery, for example removing fibroids.

I've included below a sample scenario that gives you a glimpse of what you can expect from your initial consult. It will enable you to understand how jarring the initial consult can be for some who might not be prepared. I will call the patients Mary and Tim. This is their first time going into an infertility program.

Mary and Tim have been married for three years. She is 32 and Tim is 33. They have decided to start a family. Mary's cycle can be off sometimes and she has very heavy menstrual cycles. There are months that Mary misses her menstrual cycles and there are months where she bleeds for almost three weeks out of the month.

Mary has already discussed with her gynecologist that she wants to get pregnant. Her OB-GYN told her to get an ovulation kit from the pharmacy and start testing on day nine or 10 of her cycle (assuming a 28-day cycle). (The testing day will vary depending on the length of an individual's cycle). The ovulation kit uses urine to monitor the LH (Luteinizing hormone) surge. The patient is most likely to get pregnant when she has intercourse 24 to 36 hours after the LH surge. Ovulation kits have enough strips to test for a week and she will most likely test for six to seven days. It is best to test the same time of the day either in the morning or afternoon, be consistent.

Mary's OB-GYN told her that if she didn't get pregnant after first trying the ovulation kit for six months to a year, to set up a follow-up appointment to consult with an infertility specialist. After trying for seven months and not getting pregnant, Mary took the next step and made an appointment with the specialist. Right off the bat, she was told by the office to check with her insurance company on infertility benefits (as noted in chapter 2). The office also indicated that they request from her gynecologist any records that would help the specialist at this stage.

On the day of the consult Mary and Tim were checked in to fill out the preliminary paperwork regarding her medical history. The reproductive specialist (RE) greeted them and introduced himself, then they walked together to the consult room. After discussing Mary's medical history (her cycles and how long they have been trying) and asking Tim if he has ever had a semen analysis, he then asked the couple if they had any questions or concerns.

Mary asked the first question that is typically asked by most women at this stage:

What are our chances of getting pregnant? The doctor indicated that some lab tests would need to be performed for both her and Tim before he can answer that question satisfactorily. He did indicate that at her age now, he felt she had a good chance of a successful pregnancy. Mary also asked about the chances of multiple births. The doctor assured her it was a common question. He indicated that a patient delivering twins, or even triplets, is not uncommon, but that it was his job to monitor Mary's response to the treatment and to prevent her from having, as he put it, "a litter."[38]

Once the questions had been asked and answered, the doctor introduced Mary to her nurse who will work with her to organize the treatments. This will be the main nurse that she will converse with over the phone and to whom she should request to speak to with ongoing questions when Mary calls. The nurse will navigate the couple through the process of making appointments for testing, and the follow-up second consult that takes place when the testing is completed in approximately three months.

Mary and Tim then spoke to one of the nurses who gave them a packet of instructions for testing. One of the first test almost every woman is tested for in the infertility program is the Clomid Challenge Test (CCT) which checks your ovarian function and ovarian reserve. The CCT checks a blood sample on days three and 10 of Mary's cycle. She will take the medication Clomid on days five through nine. The nurse needs to know exactly when Mary has reached day three of her menstrual cycle, so the patient calls the nurse on the first day of her period, which is the first day of a complete flow, not merely spotting. This way, the nurse can schedule Mary for a day-three blood work up. The nurse will also give you a prescription for Clomid that you will have to fill at your pharmacy. There should be an instruction sheet in your packet, which explains more, and I explain further in Chapter 9. Then the nurse gave Tim a specimen cup along with an instruction sheet for a semen analysis and instructed him to call the lab to book the appointment. (Telling him the lab would review all the instructions with him.)

Until Mary's menstrual cycle begins, the nurse indicated there is nothing more to be done. Once she called on day one, they would prepare for the blood work to be drawn on day three.[39]

About three weeks from the Initial appointment:

Mary called her nurse on the first day of her menstrual cycle, which meant she could do the CCT. The nurse reviewed the instructions with Mary telling her to come on Day three for blood work, after which she would take Clomid (on days five through nine). Then, she would come back in on day 10 for another blood test. At this time her nurse had booked the second, follow up appointment with the RE and asked if Tim had already had his semen analysis. Mary said Tim had called the lab and booked the semen analysis earlier that week.

When Tim called the lab to book the semen analysis, the lab technician indicated that the optimal time to take a specimen was after two to four days of abstinence. They instructed him, as well, to keep the specimen against his body while transporting it and that the specimen should be delivered within 45 minutes from time of collection. If he felt it might take longer, the lab suggested collecting the specimen at the center.

Chapter 8
Female & Male Reproductive Systems

It is important to understand what goes on inside our bodies and to realize how complicated the female and male reproductive systems are. This is the only way to explore and understand which different areas may not be working properly and can cause infertility. I am compelled to add that, as complicated as it is, most times everything works just fine and it is amazing how the end product is a beautiful baby.

How well do you remember high school biology?

A woman is born with all of the eggs that she will ever have. A newborn baby girl has up to 400,000 eggs stored in the ovaries. During a woman's reproductive years, a total of about 400 eggs are released. At puberty, a woman begins to have menstrual cycles, which enables her to release from one of her ovaries an egg each month. Each menstrual cycle begins on the first day of menstrual flow to the first day of her next flow. As each new cycle begins, a new egg starts to grow. After two weeks (depending on 28 day cycle) a mature egg (ovum) is released from the ovary and is picked up by one of the fallopian tubes where it is positioned to be fertilized by one of the many sperm that may surround it.

If the egg is fertilized it will implant in the uterine wall. The placenta forms between the uterus and the newly growing embryo. The placenta and the umbilical cord bring oxygen and nutrients to the embryo from the mother and takes away waste from embryo to the placenta. The embryo will grow into a healthy baby.

If the egg does not get fertilized then the egg will leave the body in about two weeks during the female menstrual cycle.

What's a normal menstrual cycle?[40]

An average menstrual cycle lasts approximately 28 days, counting from the first day of one period to the day before the next. There are two phases in the menstrual cycle: the follicular stage, from day one to day 14 (when ovulation should occur); and the luteal phase, from day 14 to day 28, when the fertilized egg implants in the uterus. Some women have shorter cycles, lasting only 23 days; some have much longer ones, lasting up to 35 days. If your cycle is shorter or longer this could indicate a hormonal problem, so it might be beneficial to consult your OB-GYN.

Your menstrual cycle is controlled by many hormones produced in various parts of the body. Getting to know their names and their respective jobs will help you understand what is being monitored when you have your blood drawn and what your RE is looking at during a stimulation cycle.

The female ovulation cycle includes the following hormonal elements and interactions:

- *Gonadotropin Releasing Hormone (GnRH)*: produced by the hypothalamus in the brain
- *Follicle Stimulating Hormone (FSH)*: produced by the pituitary gland in the brain
- *Luteinizing Hormone* (LH): produced by the pituitary gland
- *Estrogen:* produced by the ovaries
- *Progesterone:* produced by the ovaries

The cycle begins when the hypothalamus produces GnRH, which travels to the pituitary gland and signals it to release follicle-stimulating hormone (FSH). FSH stimulates the ovaries to start ripening eggs. The eggs are in little sacs called follicles. One follicle, or possibly two, will start growing faster than the others.

FSH also stimulates the ovaries to produce estrogen, which enables the eggs to mature and at the same time starts thickening the uterine lining, preparing it to support a pregnancy if the egg is fertilized.

Ovulation: the egg is released

Approximately mid-cycle, the LH surges and this triggers ovulation. (This is the hormone being measured in the over-the-counter ovulation kits.) At ovulation the mature egg is released from the follicle and is caught by the fallopian tubes and starts its travel down the tube.

Normally your cervix (the neck of your uterus) is closed

and is only opened during ovulation and menstrual bleeding. Just before ovulation the cervical mucus becomes thin and stretchy which allows the sperm to swim through the cervix into the uterus and up the fallopian tubes to meet with the egg.

After ovulation

The empty follicle that released the egg collapses and becomes corpus luteum. The corpus luteum produces the hormone progesterone, which acts on the lining of the uterus to become thick and spongy getting it ready for implantation. As progesterone rises, your breasts may feel larger and sore. The pituitary gland stops producing FSH so that eggs will not continue to mature in your ovaries.

The released egg will fertilize in the fallopian tube, and it will move down to the uterus, where it will implant in the lining. This takes about five days. The progesterone levels will stay high and you may start to feel the early signs of pregnancy such as tenderness in the breasts, feeling fatigue, and feeling nausea are just some symptoms. The embryo produces Human Chorionic Gonadotropin (HCG), which is the "pregnancy hormone" that is measured by a blood sample to see if you are pregnant. It is also produced in the urine, which is tested by means of over-the-counter pregnancy kits.

If the egg isn't fertilized or does not successfully implant, it will start to disintegrate and the corpus luteum shrinks. The estrogen and progesterone levels drop and the lining of your uterus will shed, becoming your menstrual flow. The uterus will be replaced with a new lining on the next month.

How do I test to see if I'm ovulating?

Women who maintain a regular 28-day cycle should ovulate around day 14 or 15 of the cycle. Some common symptoms of ovulation are cramps, tenderness in the breasts, and vaginal discharge. Some women may not even know when they are ovulating, to determine how many days are in your cycle, count day one as the first day of your period (full flow of bleeding) and the last day of your cycle is the day before your next period. So if your period began on January 1 and you next period began on January 31st.[41] The last day is the day before, which would be January 30th, so you have a 30-day cycle. There is always a fertile window of five to six days. The sperm can stay viable up to five days before ovulation and fertilization can occur up to 24 hours after ovulation. Everyone's cycle is different and it is sometimes hard to predict. When you are serious about getting pregnant you must mark your calendar to keep track of your cycle. Mark your calendar on day one of your menstrual cycle (day one is full flow) and watch to see if it is consistent each month.[42]

Ovulation Predictor Kits

Ovulation Prediction Kits (OPK) are a very popular method of detecting ovulation. These can be purchased in local drug stores or on-line. One of the benefits of using an OPK is that you can predict ovulation before it occurs. The kits work by detecting LH (Luteinizing Hormone) levels in your urine. The hormone will increase or spike just before ovulation and you should ovulate approximately 36 hours after this spike. You usually start testing on day nine or 10 of your cycle (you may want to ask your OB-GYN or infertility nurse on what day to start). This test is very similar to a pregnancy test in which you test your urine mid-stream or dip the stick into your urine sample (depending on the type of OPK). Then, according to the instructions, read the test results within a certain time period (usually five minutes). A control line will appear to ensure that the kit is working properly. The test line should be the same color as the control line, if not darker, to register a positive result. It is best to test your urine the same time everyday either in the morning or late afternoon.[43]

When you are in an infertility program, your nurse will suggest that you purchase ovulation kits and start testing around day nine of your cycle. They usually suggest testing in the late afternoon, before 5:00 p.m., so that if the kit turns positive, you can call your nurse and get your instructions on what to do next (depending on your specific course of fertility treatment).

Monitoring Cervical Mucus Changes

Cervical Mucus (CM) is produced by the cervix and is stimulated by the hormone estrogen. During your menstrual cycle, the amount and quality of the cervical mucus changes, as you get closer to your fertile time. (Some women can tell when they are ovulating by the presence of cervical mucus.) How amazing is the whole process of conception that changes the mucus during your fertile period to aid the sperm on its journey to the egg! When it's not your fertile time the mucus goes to a consistency that inhibits the sperm. As your cycle progresses the mucus changes to a sticky white or cream-colored discharge. As it gets closer to ovulation the mucus will resemble egg white color and consistency.[44] After ovulation the mucus subsides to little or none, which is dry or sticky.[45]

Basal Body Temperature[46]

Growing up my mom told me I was a "basal thermometer baby." I have finally come to understand what that meant. The basal body temperature (BBT) is the lowest temperature of the body during rest, usually during sleep. It is usually measured first in the morning after awakening before any physical activity occurs. In women, ovulation causes an increase of one-half to one degree Fahrenheit (one-quarter to one-half degree Celsius) in basal body temperature. Monitoring the BBT is one way to calculate the day of ovulation. The basal thermometer is ultra-sensitive and is able to measure the slightest change in the basal temperature. (Now that the thermometer is digital it is even easier to read.) Women take their temperature using a basal thermometer while they are still in bed and track it on a chart. It's best to take it the same time everyday, so setting an alarm clock will help. (The basal charts are available at the drug stores.) Each reading must be recorded. You will see a rise in temperature when you have ovulated. As each day's temperature is plotted on the graph, you will learn to recognize your own pattern. Your temperature rise may be sudden, gradual, or incremental. The pattern may vary from cycle to cycle. The temperature can rise from 0.4 degrees F up to 0.8 degrees F before, during or right after ovulation.

You must also realize that your BBT can be influenced by physical or emotional upsets, or even the lack of sleep. In addition, illness, emotional distress, jet lag, disturbed sleep, smoking, drinking an unaccustomed amount of alcohol the night before, and using an electric blanket may affect your body temperature. Noting such events on the chart helps to interpret the readings.

BBT charting is quite accurate in detecting when ovulation has occurred. Even so, it cannot predict when it's about to happen. The ovulation predictor kit serves that end, turning positive just before ovulation. Some patients use both BBT and OPK simultaneously. Charting your temperature for several months will allow you to better pinpoint your ovulation and, in turn, time intercourse before ovulation, increasing your chances of getting pregnant.

Sperm generally remain capable of fertilizing an egg for two to three days after ejaculation. There are even instances of sperm remaining active five or more days after intercourse. So if you have sexual intercourse several days before ovulation, there's a good chance that live sperm could still fertilize a newly released egg.

The Male Reproductive System:[47]

The purpose of the organs of the male reproductive system is to perform the following functions:

- To produce, maintain, and transport sperm (the male reproductive cells) and protective fluid (semen)
- To discharge sperm within the female reproductive tract during sex
- To produce and secrete male sex hormones responsible for maintaining the male reproductive system

Unlike the female reproductive system, most of the male reproductive system is located outside of the body. These external structures include the penis, scrotum, and testicles.

Penis: This is the male organ used in sexual intercourse. It has three parts: the root, which attaches to the wall of the abdomen the body, or shaft; and the glans, which is the cone-shaped part at the end of the penis. The glans, also called the head of the penis, is covered with a loose layer of skin called foreskin. This skin is sometimes removed in a procedure called circumcision. The opening of the urethra, the tube that transports semen and urine, is at the tip of the penis. The penis also contains a number of sensitive nerve endings.

The body of the penis is cylindrical in shape and consists of three circular shaped chambers. These chambers are made up of special, sponge-like tissue. This tissue contains thousands of large spaces that fill with blood when the man is sexually aroused. As the penis fills with blood, it becomes rigid and erect, which allows for penetration during sexual intercourse. The skin of the penis is loose and elastic to accommodate changes in penis size during an erection.

Semen, which contains sperm (reproductive cells), is expelled (ejaculated) through the end of the penis when the man reaches sexual climax (orgasm). When the penis is erect, the flow of urine is blocked from the urethra, allowing only semen to be ejaculated at orgasm.

Scrotum: This is the loose pouch-like sac of skin that hangs behind and below the penis. It contains the testicles (also called testes), as well as many nerves and blood vessels. The scrotum acts as a "climate control system" for the testes. For normal sperm development, the testes must be at a temperature slightly cooler than body temperature. Special muscles in the wall of the scrotum allow it to contract and relax, moving the testicles closer to the body for warmth or farther away from the body to cool the temperature.

Testicles (testes): These are oval organs about the size of large olives that lie in the scrotum, secured at either end by a structure called the spermatic cord. Most men have two testes. The testes are responsible for making testosterone, the primary male sex hormone, and for generating sperm. Within the testes are coiled masses of tubes called seminiferous tubules. These tubes are responsible for producing sperm cells.

The internal organs of the male reproductive system,

also called accessory organs, include the following:

Epididymis: The epididymis is a long, coiled tube that rests on the backside of each testicle. It transports and stores sperm cells that are produced in the testes. It also is the job of the epididymis to bring the sperm to maturity, since the sperm that emerge from the testes are immature and incapable of fertilization. During sexual arousal, contractions force the sperm into the vas deferens.

Vas deferens: The vas deferens is a long, muscular tube that travels from the epididymis into the pelvic cavity, to just behind the bladder. The vas deferens transports mature sperm to the urethra, the tube that carries urine or sperm to outside of the body, in preparation for ejaculation. Some men are missing these vas deferens, so they are not producing any sperm. There is a procedure where the doctor can remove epididymis tissue where the sperm are maturing there and these can be used for IVF.

Ejaculatory ducts: These are formed by the fusion of the vas deferens and the seminal vesicles. The ejaculatory ducts empty into the urethra.

Urethra: The urethra is the tube that carries urine from the bladder to outside of the body. In males, it has the additional function of ejaculating semen when the man reaches orgasm. When the penis is erect during sex, the flow of urine is blocked from the urethra, allowing only semen to be ejaculated at orgasm.

Seminal vesicles: The seminal vesicles are sac-like pouches that attach to the vas deferens near the base of the bladder. The seminal vesicles produce a sugar-rich fluid (fructose) that provides sperm with a source of energy to help them move. The fluid of the seminal vesicles makes up most of the volume of a man's ejaculatory fluid, or ejaculate.

Prostate gland: The prostate gland is a walnut-sized structure that is located below the urinary bladder in front of the rectum. The prostate gland contributes additional fluid to the ejaculate. Prostate fluids also help to nourish the sperm. The urethra, which carries the ejaculate to be expelled during orgasm, runs through the center of the prostate gland.

Bulbourethral glands: Also called Cowper's glands, these are pea-sized structures located on the sides of the urethra just below the prostate gland. These glands produce a clear, slippery fluid that empties directly into the urethra. This fluid serves to lubricate the urethra and to neutralize any acidity that may be present due to residual drops of urine in the urethra.

How Does the Male Reproductive System Function?

The entire male reproductive system is dependent on hormones, which are chemicals that regulate the activity of many different types of cells or organs. The primary hormones involved in the male reproductive system are follicle-stimulating hormone, luteinizing hormone, and testosterone.

Follicle-stimulating hormone (FSH) is necessary for sperm production (spermatogenesis) and luteinizing hormone (LH) stimulates the production of testosterone, which is also needed to make sperm. Testosterone is responsible for the development of male characteristics, including muscle mass and strength, fat distribution, bone mass, facial hair growth, voice change, and sex drive.

Don't Worry

Wow. Here you thought the female reproductive system was confusing! You can see that we all, males and females, possess the same hormones, only in different quantities. Both female and male reproductive systems are very complex, but well understood by infertility specialists and urologists. So don't worry if something is not quite right or you aren't clear on something. Once you go to the professionals who know your situation, they will help you both as a couple.

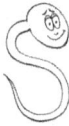

panky is bringing a patient
to the collection room
and the patient says,
"Is room service included?"

Chapter 9
Female Testing

There are a couple of diagnostic tests the specialist may order on the female, called a Hysteroscopy and a Hysterosalpingogram (HSG). A hysteroscopy looks at the lining of the uterus and is best performed after your menstrual cycle when the uterus is thin. This is a simple procedure performed in the office using a local anesthesia. A narrow thin microscope, called a hysteroscope, passes through the cervix to examine the uterus for fibroids, polyps or other problems that could cause bleeding. You may be told to take Tylenol before the procedure to help with cramping.

The second test, a HSG, is performed in the X-ray department of your medical facility and looks for blockages or debris in the fallopian tubes. The X-ray creates a picture of the uterus and fallopian tubes into which colored dye has been injected into the vagina through the uterus and travels up into the fallopian tubes. Pictures can be taken as the dye flows through and blockages can be identified. A blockage in the fallopian tube could stop the sperm from passing through the tubes to the egg. Some patients have said this procedure can be uncomfortable.

The specialist will order blood work, which may include

measuring the following hormones: Follicle-Stimulating Hormone (FSH), E2 (estradiol), Prolactin, Progesterone and Thyroid-Stimulating Hormone (TSH). Hormones control many functions of the body, including your menstrual cycle, fertility, maintaining pregnancy, weight gain or weight loss. The medical team will also undertake genetic testing for possible complications such as cystic fibrosis and Sexually Transmitted Diseases (STDs).

The level of FSH on day three of a normal menstrual cycle is a critical prognostic indicator for a women considering Assisted Reproductive Technologies (ART). In a normal menstrual cycle FSH levels rise and fall predictably and are used by the specialist, along with other tests, to predict accurately the ovulation stimulation response and probability of pregnancy. One test that the RE will perform is called the Clomid Challenge Test (CCT).

The Clomid Challenge Test (CCT) measures ovarian function and ovarian reserve. During this test you call the nurse on the first day of your menstrual cycle. The first day is considered the first day of a full flow, not early spotting. So if your period commences with spotting wait until you have a full flow. That is considered day one.

The nurse will have you come in on day three of your cycle and have your blood drawn for FSH testing. You'll then be given a medication called clomiphene to take on days five through nine of your cycle. (A prescription will be given the day of your consult.) You will then return on day 10 of your cycle for a second FSH blood draw. When the physician gets both results he can compare the results of your FSH levels on days three and ten, this will enable your doctor to get a clear understanding of your ovarian reserve or ovarian failure (depending upon FSH values). The physician likes to see the day-three FSH levels on the low side. Every clinic or lab uses different kits or assays to test for FSH, so a result of 12 could mean "good" ovarian reserve where at another lab a 12 could mean "fair" ovarian reserve.

A poor Clomid Challenge Test (CCT) or a high day-three FSH often indicates a decreased response to ovarian stimulation and that the pregnancy success rates will be lessened and that there is an increased chance of miscarriage. In younger women (35 and under) the high FSH levels are often indicative of decreased ovarian function. Even so, options such as IVF are often still successful. In women over 35 and certainly over 40 years old, an elevated FSH or abnormal (CCT) indicates chances for successful pregnancy are often less than ten percent. In this case the physician will use the acronym "DOR," which stands for Diminished Ovarian Reserve. In that circumstance, some couples choose instead a donor egg program because of its high success rates. Your RE will explain these results and review the options available.

There is one more test that a specialist may perform: a postcoital test. A postcoital test checks a woman's cervical mucus after sex to see whether sperm are present and moving normally. This test may be used if tests have not found a measurable cause for not conceiving. The test is done one to two days before ovulation when the cervical mucus is thin and stretchy and sperm can easily move through it into the uterus. Within two to eight hours after intercourse your doctor collects and looks at a cervical mucus sample for the presence of motile sperm.[48]

Chapter 10
Recurrent Miscarriage

Recurrent miscarriage, or habitual pregnancy loss, is defined as three or more consecutive, spontaneous pregnancy losses. Many reproductive endocrinologists will begin looking into the cause at the point at which a woman has experienced at least two consecutive miscarriages.

Possible causes include a genetic defect that can come from the egg, sperm or the early embryo, an abnormally shaped uterus, uterine fibroids, scar tissue, hormonal imbalances or illness such as diabetes. Life style habits can also increase a woman's risk for miscarriage. These include smoking, caffeine, alcohol, and the use of certain medications.

The RE will take a detailed medical, family and genetic history of the couple. A karyotype may be drawn on the couple. A karyotype is a blood test, which shows the genetic makeup of a person. The medical workup for this problem usually involves blood work. Each specialist among the entire ART team undertakes a panel of tests, some drawn from the female and some drawn from the male. The majority of the workup for the recurrent miscarriage is done on the female consisting of more blood work and a complete physical.

Age is also a significant factor that could account for recurrent miscarriage in women. Women 35 or older not only are battling infertility issues generally, but also contend with a higher risk of recurrent miscarriage. The RE will perform the following tests to diagnose recurrent miscarriage:

- Hormone levels and diabetes
- Chromosomes of both partners depending on genetic history and ethnicity
- Uterine Abnormalities, specifically a uterine septum (a wall that divides the uterus into 2 parts), which would cause problems in implantation. There could be uterine fibroids also present.
- Antiphospholipid Syndrome. Your body has a defense mechanism to produce antibodies to fight any invaders, such as bacteria or virus. Sometimes the immune system doesn't function properly and produces antibodies against tissues in its own body. These antibodies work against phospholipids to stimulate blood clots and cause miscarriage. The female will have blood work drawn for the Antiphospholipid antibody, lupus anticoagulant and other tests in this category.[49]
- Asherman's Syndrome. This is a term used to describe the presence of scar tissues (adhesions) between opposing endometrial (uterine) surfaces inside the uterine cavity. The adhesions can be mild or severe, causing significant damage to the

uterus. Scar tissue in this area can interfere with implantation of the embryo from an IVF treatment, as well as increase the risk of miscarriage. Causes for this syndrome can be the result of surgical procedures performed on the uterus (removal of fibroids) or Pelvic Inflammatory Disease (PID) infection in the uterus.[50]

There is a specific gene found on a chromosome, which produces an enzyme to convert an amino acid homocysteine to another amino acid methionine, which are used to make other proteins in the body. This is called Methylenetetrahydrofolate reductase (MTHFR). If there is an abnormal change in this gene, called a mutation, this can disrupt the production of homocysteine. Some women who have had multiple miscarriages have been shown to have the MTHFR gene mutation. Whether or not the MTHFR gene mutation is directly linked to recurrent pregnancy loss remains under debate. Your specialist will be able to guide you and clarify questions you may possess regarding the necessity of this test. [51]

Evidence has also emerged that certain sperm DNA may cause miscarriage. The male may have his semen tested for DNA fragmentation, which is a fairly new test.

Depending on the findings of your RE, treatments for these symptoms are available. These include medications for hormonal abnormalities, possible some uterine surgery to correct the septum, removal of fibroids, taking an aspirin for blood clots and other advanced ART procedures for abnormal sperm. It should be noted however that there is a certain percentage of miscarriages that simply remained unexplained. After all testing is completed, 50 to 75 percent of couples with recurrent pregnancy loss come to no definitive explanation as to why their pregnancies don't go to term. Still, studies have also shown that these couples still have a 60 percent probability of producing a live birth.

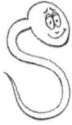

panky pointed out the collection room
to a patient, and the patient said:
"Is there a beautiful woman in there?"
And Spanky said, "Yes, she is in a magazine!"

Chapter 11
Causes of Female Infertility
& Sexually Transmitted Diseases

There are many causes of female infertility. A woman has to ovulate to become pregnant and for some women, ovulation disorders predispose them to infertility. Age is the most pronounced reason for problems conceiving if the female is 35 years or older. Beyond that, several other factors can cause for infertility in females, which are explored below.

Ovulation Disorder

Ovulation Disorders mean an inability to release an egg or that the egg not being released at the right time in the cycle to cause conception. Ovulation Disorders can be characterized by anovulation (absent ovulation), which results in infrequent periods (oligomenorrhea). Several additional different factors can cause Ovulation Disorders. These include:

- Hormone imbalances
- Hyperthyroidism (Low TSH)
- Hypothyroidism (High TSH)
- Low body weight or Body Mass Index (BMI)
- High body weight or high BMI

- Smoking and the use of illicit drugs (marijuana, narcotics and cocaine)[52]
- Luteal Phase Defect (LPD): the luteal phase is the period of (normally) 14 days[53] in a woman's cycle between ovulation and menstruation. If a woman is pregnant, during the luteal phase the fertilized egg will travel from the fallopian tube and into the uterus for implantation. If your luteal phase lasts under 10 days it is considered a luteal phase defect.[54]

Ovulation disorders, for women who are trying to conceive, create additional complications when it comes to their chances of conceiving because it is difficult to determine when exactly they are ovulating.

Hormones

Our bodies have many feedback loops that determine how much of each hormone is to be present and when they are to be present.[55] This ongoing communication travels back and forth among the brain, the ovaries and the adrenal glands. If the concentration of one or more of the hormones is too low or too high it affects the feedback loop, disrupts communication between these vital entities and sabotages the normal course for ovulation.

Undiagnosed and untreated thyroid disease can cause infertility or recurrent miscarriage. The thyroid hormone is important for growth and metabolism, and because it regulates cellular function, abnormal thyroid function can affect your fertility. Thyroid Stimulating Hormone (TSH) is usually checked for any evidence of thyroid disease, which is common among females. A low level of TSH is seen in hyperthyroid patients that have an overactive thyroid gland and a high TSH is seen with hypothyroid patients that have an underactive thyroid gland. Either condition may cause fertility problems because both cause hormonal imbalances, leading to ovulations disorders and other problems in the menstrual cycle.

Prolactin is a hormone that is produced by the pituitary gland in pregnant women to bring on milk production for nursing. When prolactin is being produced, FSH and gonadotropin-releasing hormone (GnRH) (the hormones that stimulate the ovaries to produce and mature eggs for ovulation) stop production. This is why you may have heard that you cannot get pregnant while you are nursing.[56] Some patients (approximately 10 percent) might have what is called Prolactinoma, a tumor on their pituitary gland, which increases prolactin production – hence, stopping ovulation. These tumors usually do not pose any serious health risks other than affecting fertility. Typically your RE will draw a prolactin level on the first visit with your other hormones. If the prolactin is elevated the RE may ask the patient to return and have a fasting prolactin drawn, which is a more accurate test. Prolactin can be increased after a high protein meal. A fasting blood draw means nothing has been eaten for 12 to 14 hours prior to having blood taken.[57]

Progesterone is the hormone that prepares the body for pregnancy. It is produced by the corpus luteum, which is what remains of the collapsed ovarian follicle once ovulation takes place. Once the egg is released from the follicle (ovulation) the ovarian follicle becomes corpus luteum and begins to produce progesterone. The increase in progesterone builds the uterine lining and gets the uterus ready for implantation of the fertilized egg. Progesterone levels rise just after ovulation and will stay elevated to support the uterus for implantation and the pregnancy. Its staying elevated prevents another menstrual cycle. If there is no pregnancy then progesterone levels drop, which then triggers the next menstrual cycle. The increase in progesterone occurs during the luteal phase, which is the period of time from ovulation to menstruation, normally lasting 14 days. A luteal phase defect is a shorter period of time in the second half of the cycle. If it is, say, 10 days, it may indicate a potential problem with the production of progesterone.

The body starts naturally to decrease progesterone in women in their thirties and forties, so this is one test that your RE will test for. You'll learn later in the book that when you are in an IVF cycle the increase in progesterone after you ovulate is the starting point for the IVF cycle.

As previously noted, your RE will have blood drawn to test the following hormones: FSH, LH, E2, Prolactin, Progesterone, Testosterone and TSH. These encompass the scope of probable hormonal disorders.

Subsequent treatment depends upon the diagnosis. It may include fertility medications (oral and injectables), nutritional changes, and surgery (for tumors or cysts). Hormonal problems can be treated with medications, which will regulate ovulation in 90 percent of women.

Weight

Weight plays a major role with infertility. Body Mass Index or BMI is a tool used to measure the amount of body fat based on your weight and height. It is an overall indicator physicians use to evaluate a person's general health status.[58]

A normal BMI range falls between 18.5 and 24.9. (You may see slight variations.) The former, 18.5 and below is considered underweight, whereas a BMI range of 25 to 29.9 is considered over weight. A BMI of more than 30 is considered obese.

A low weight can cause a disruption in the hormone levels making it difficult to conceive. Women who are very athletic with very low BMI can skip their menstrual cycles or not get them at all. A women's body is built to bear children and it needs body fat to do this. When the weight is so low the body goes into a starvation mode and everything stops including, the possibility of getting pregnant, because your body is in a defense mode. Under this kind of duress, the body would not be able to carry a pregnancy. If you do conceive with a low BMI there is a higher risk for miscarriage and low birth weight for the child.

A high BMI can also cause hormonal problems, which affects ovulation. In this instance, you are less likely to conceive without medical intervention and you remain at higher risk for miscarriage and pregnancy complications, such as early delivery.

Some insurance companies will not cover infertility treatments for those who have a very high BMI. Or, in some cases, if a patient possesses a BMI greater than or equal to 40, she may need to show documentation that she is seeing a nutritionist and fulfilling other requirements for coverage.

I had a patient in our program that left temporarily to take a break. When she returned she had gained weight and the guidelines for infertility protocols had changed. She told me she would have to lose weight before she could continue further treatment. The insurance companies know the problems and risks factors that go along with a high BMI and are not going to pay for it.

Pelvic Inflammatory Disease

Pelvic inflammatory disease (PID) is a general term for infection and inflammation of the female reproductive system. PID occurs when bacteria move from the vagina or cervix into the uterus, fallopian tubes, ovaries, or pelvis. If the infection progresses undetected it produces scar tissue to the nearby tissues and organs, which in turn form adhesions. Adhesions are abnormal bands of scar tissue that join together organs or parts of organs that aren't meant to be connected. In most cases PID is caused by the sexually transmitted diseases (STDs) gonorrhea and chlamydia. The problem with PID as it relates to infertility is that in some women it is asymptomatic (no symptoms). The infection can affect their organs to the extent that they can become infertile. Although STDs are often the cause of PID, the bacteria can enter the body through other means such as childbirth, insertion of an IUD, miscarriage, or an elective or therapeutic abortion. A pelvic ultrasound is a procedure that is be done to diagnosis PID to determine if the fallopian tubes are enlarged. In some cases a laparoscopy is necessary to confirm the diagnosis. A laparoscopy is a surgical procedure during which a thin, rigid tube with a camera is inserted into the abdomen through a small incision. This enables the physician to view the pelvic organs and look for any abnormalities. Because PID is asymptomatic, women who have had laparoscopic procedures for other reasons have been found to have PID who were otherwise unaware of it.[59]

According to the CDC, each year in the United States, it is estimated that more than 750,000 women experience an episode of acute PID. Up to 10 to 15 percent of these women may become infertile as a result. A large proportion of the ectopic pregnancies occur every year that are directly related to the effects of PID.[60]

Common symptoms include fever, chills, pain or tenderness in the pelvic region, vaginal discharge with an abnormal color and odor. Other symptoms may include pain during intercourse or bleeding after intercourse, frequent and painful urination, increased menstrual pain and bleeding or no menstrual cycle at all. If you possess any of these symptoms, your doctor will perform a pelvic exam and may do blood work, vaginal and or cervical cultures for the STDs. Mild cases can be treated with antibiotics but more severe cases may require a hospital stay. Sexual partners must be treated to prevent infection from being passed back and forth. Complicated cases where antibiotics are not working may require surgery.

Serious cases, especially if left untreated, can cause scarring of the pelvic organs and lead to chronic pelvic pain, ectopic pregnancy and infertility because of the damage to the fallopian tubes and other organs.

If you have any symptoms or feel you may have an STD please contact your physician as soon as possible.

Polycystic Ovary Syndrome

Polycystic Ovary Syndrome (PCOS) is a very common condition affecting five to ten percent of women. It occurs when there is an imbalance of hormones that regulate the menstruation cycle and cause a failure to ovulate. The imbalance also shows itself in the increase of the male hormones, called androgens (including testosterone). As androgens increase certain symptoms appear, acne, excessive hair growth and irregular or missed menses. Some women may have irregular heavy bleeding. The ovary contains follicles, which are sacs that contain an egg. Normally, one or more eggs are released during each menstrual cycle. With PCOS the eggs in these follicles do not mature and are not released from the ovaries. Instead, they form very small cysts in the ovary. These changes can contribute to infertility.

Women are usually diagnosed when in their twenties or thirties, but PCOS may also affect teenage girls. The symptoms often begin when a girl's periods start. Women with this disorder often have a mother or sister who have had similar symptoms. If you have PCOS you should see your doctor every six to 12 months. This is because; if you have PCOS you are not ovulating nor producing the hormone progesterone, which works with estrogen to build up the lining of your uterus. Many times, this condition can be treated with medications such as contraceptive pills or anti-androgen therapy. The most important treatment, however, begins with the patient tending to her general health, including weight loss. I know of a woman who had PCOS and after she lost 30 pounds, suddenly got her menstrual cycle back on track without medical intervention. The importance of maintaining a healthy body weight for optimal body function cannot be overstated. Often you'll find that, with a corrected body weight your body kicks back into action![61]

Patients with PCOS may be given a trial of Clomiphene (Clomid is an infertility drug used to induce ovulation) to attempt to induce ovulation. The patient would be monitored for development of follicles. If unsuccessful, the RE may recommend FSH gonadotropin (hormone) injections. The patient would typically be given a low dose over a lengthy stretch of 7 to 14 days, being monitored closely to determine how many follicles and/or eggs develop. In some instances, women with PCOS respond too exuberantly, meaning they developed too many follicles. In this case their IUI treatment for that particular month would be canceled to avoid multiple pregnancies.

Many women with PCOS exhibit insulin resistance and have a higher risk of diabetes. This type of diabetes is more commonly associated with obesity but it has likewise been seen in women of normal weight who have PCOS. Insulin resistance is a condition where the cells fail to respond to insulin. Insulin's job is to regulate the delivery of sugar into the cells, which is needed for energy. A recent study determined that up to 40 percent of obese reproductive-age women with PCOS had impaired glucose tolerance and 7.5 percent had diabetes. In addition, 15 percent of normal-weight women with PCOS had impaired glucose tolerance and 1.5 percent had diabetes, a rate almost three-times that of the general population. If untreated, insulin resistance leads to diabetes in approximately one-third of patients.[62]

Endometriosis

Endometriosis refers to a condition that can be an extremely painful disease in which cells from the lining of the uterus, called the endometrium, break away and migrate to other parts of the body. This tissue can grow on the ovaries, lining of the abdominal cavity, fallopian tubes, bladder, intestines or the space between the uterus and rectum. Occasionally these cells can invade the lungs, brain, armpits and legs. Because the tissue is made up of the endometrium (mucous membrane lining of the uterus), these growths respond to hormonal changes of the menstrual cycle. These hormonal changes will build them up and break them down monthly just as the uterus does. The result is internal bleeding, inflammation, formation of blood-filled cysts, and scar tissue (known as adhesions). This causes the patient chronic pelvic pain.[63]

Endometriosis affects five million women in the United States and 30 to 40 percent of women with endometriosis are infertile. Women are infertile because these pelvic adhesions prevent the fallopian tubes from capturing the egg or the adhesions could be preventing the ovaries in releasing the egg. The cause of endometriosis is unknown, although one theory posits it is a result of a condition called "reverse menstruation." Whereas most menstrual flow leaves the uterus by way of the cervix, sometime a small amount may go up the fallopian tube and enter the abdominal cavity. This "reverse menstruation" can possibly set the stage for endometriosis.

It is important to remember that having endometriosis does not automatically mean that you will never have children. Rather, it means that you may have more difficulties getting pregnant and should be aware of it. Many women with endometriosis have children without difficulty, and many others become pregnant eventually – though it may take time, and may require the help of surgery or assisted reproductive technologies or both.

The most common symptom of endometriosis is pelvic pain. Other symptoms include mild to extreme pain before, during or after the menstrual period; pain during bowel movements or urination; pain during sex; bleeding from unusual places (such as the rectum) during the menstrual period; nausea and vomiting during the menstrual period; and infertility. Sometimes there are no symptoms and it may be discovered only during an infertility exam.

Endometriosis symptoms can be confused with other possibly conditions like, Pelvic Inflammatory Disease (PID), and irritable bowel syndrome and sometimes may be thought to be menstrual cramps. An ultrasound should be performed when there is pelvic pain. A definitive diagnosis can be made through laparoscopic surgery where the surgeon can see directly in the pelvic region and determine any endometrial growths.

Treatment usually falls into one or both categories: hormone therapy and surgery. Hormone therapy consists of birth control pills, Gonadotropin-Releasing Hormone (GnRH), and Danazol, a synthetic form of the male hormone testosterone that shrinks endometriosis tissue and reduces the pain for most women.

Hormone medication may slow the growth of endometrial implants. These hormones usually halt the menstrual cycle to allow the endometriosis to lessen but does not cure endometriosis. When this doesn't solve the problem, surgery is used to try to remove adhesions.[64]

Congenital Anomalies

Some women are born with genetic abnormalities in the reproductive system. This is called a congenital anomaly and can affect the vagina, cervix, uterus, fallopian tubes and ovaries. This can at times cause difficulty with conception or carrying a pregnancy to term. Usually an anomaly can be found during a routine Pap smear, ultrasound or laparoscopy.

Some examples of a congenital anomaly is a bicornate uterus, septae uterus and septae vagina. A bicornate uterus is known as a heart-shaped uterus where the upper part of the uterus is shaped like two horns. Pregnancies in a bicornate uterus are usually considered high-risk and require extra monitoring. A septae uterus / septae vagina is where there is a wall that divides the uterus into half and, if it goes the full length of the uterus, could cause double cervix and double vagina. Any of these maladies can lead to very painful menstrual cycles and the blockage of the outflow of blood. Correction of this involves surgery to remove the septae and it can be done hysteroscopically or through an abdominal incision (laparotomy).[65]

Uterine Fibroids

Fibroids are muscular tumors that can grow in the wall of the uterus. Fibroids are mostly benign (not cancerous) tumors. They can grow as a single or multiple tumors in the uterus, spanning in size from the size of an apple seed to a grapefruit. If a fibroid becomes too large it can affect the sperm's ability to reach the egg and cause problems with implantation in the uterus. Fibroids may be the cause of five to 10 percent of infertility cases. There is no sure cause of fibroids although estrogen levels appear to play a role in their formation. Symptoms consist of pelvic pressure or pain and irregular menstrual bleeding or spotting; urinary frequency or urgency; pressure on the abdomen; and constipation. The condition can be diagnosed through a typical pelvic examination or by means of an ultrasound. Depending on the number and size of the fibroids, they may surgically be removed before fertility treatment commences.[66]

Blocked Fallopian Tubes

The fallopian tubes are a part of the female anatomy that sweeps the egg up after it is released from the follicular sac on the ovary and passes it to the uterus. The fallopian tube is also where fertilization takes place. When the fallopian tube is blocked, it is nearly impossible for a woman to conceive since the egg and sperm cannot meet to fertilize. Since there are two fallopian tubes (one from each ovary), it is possible for one or both to become partially or totally blocked.

Sometimes tubes are blocked intentionally and other times are unintentional.

Women who chose to have their tubes blocked intentionally have a procedure called tubal ligation also known as" having their tubes tied". Once the tubes have been blocked, the chance of pregnancy is very low, unless there is failure of the procedure or if woman decides to have a reversal procedure which is called tubal reversal surgery, which will unblock the fallopian tube.

Women can have their tubes blocked unintentional and a common cause of this is scar tissue being formed either inside the tubes or outside the tubes.

The most common reasons for forming scar tissue are:

* Previous Infections - Inflammatory bowel disease
* Endometriosis

Previous infections in the pelvic region or higher in the abdomen can cause a blockage in the fallopian tube, or can cause a closure at the end of the tube or could travel across the outside of the tube. A common infection is called pelvic inflammatory disease (PID), these infections are often caused by sexually transmitted diseases, which can close the outside of the tube.

Endometriosis can cause the body's immune response to form scar tissue, which can block the tubes. Any type of pelvic surgery to the tubes, ovaries, uterus or pelvis can cause scar tissue, which can block the tubes.[67]

Testing for this includes an HSG (Hysterosalpingogram) and most specialists will order this to check for blockage. The test involves dye being injected into the uterus; pictures are taken during the time that the dye travels up the fallopian tubes. Laparoscopy can also be used to diagnose damage to the tubes. If needed, the treatment may involve tubal surgery, which is a procedure in which the physician tries to open the tube or tubes and to reduce damage to the tubes.

Sexually Transmitted Diseases and Infertility

Sexuality is an integral part of being human. Love, affection and sexual intimacy contribute to healthy relationships. But, along with the positive aspects of sexuality, there is the ongoing reality that diseases can be easily transmitted that can affect sexual health. The CDC estimates that 19 million new infections occur every year in the United States with young people between the ages of 15 and 24 (2012). Most Sexually Transmitted Diseases (STDs) are curable and treatable in the early stages. Others are asymptomatic (no symptoms) and can cause havoc in your body without realizing it. Worse, you can be spreading it to others.

STDs are infections passed from one person to another through sexual, oral, or anal intercourse; through sharing needles; mutual masturbation; or general contact with infected bodily fluids. They cause a variety of symptoms and complications, such as bumps and sores around the vagina or penis, painful urination, bleeding from vagina (other than during menstruation), pain during sex and infertility. By the age of 25, half of the sexually active adults will have an STD. If you plan on having a family it is essential to be aware of STDs and protect yourself.

It is important that you and your partner get tested for STDs and other infections, making sure you are sexually healthy. This is especially important if you are trying to get pregnant. Monitoring your sexual health will not only protect you from STDs but also prevent you from spreading it to your unborn baby. If you think you might have an STD, get tested and treated immediately. Testing involves simple blood work and an examination by a physician. This must be added to your pre-pregnancy checklist. When you start trying to have a baby you already know to watch what you eat, to take vitamins and stop drinking. You must also get your blood checked for STDs.

There are several types of STDs and associated infections that can cause serious problems. Some STDs are less serious and can be treated with a few doses of medication. Others, such as HIV/AIDS are life threatening and can cause death. If you think you may have contracted a STD it is so important to see your doctor. Treatment can usually cure STDs, or lessen the symptoms, making it less likely to spread and keeping you healthier. Get it treated immediately before it is too late.

A very common STD is chlamydia, which affects millions of men and women every year. Chlamydia is a bacterium found in vaginal fluid and semen and is transmitted through sexual intercourse. The infection spreads easily because it often doesn't show symptoms. You may be unknowingly passing it to your partner. In fact, 75 percent of infections in women and 50 percent in men show little or no symptoms. If you leave it untreated you run the risk of severe health problems, including PID, which could lead to damage of the fallopian tubes, cause infertility, and heighten the risk of an ectopic pregnancy or premature birth. The mother also can pass the infection to the child during childbirth resulting in eye infections, blindness, or pneumonia for the child. For men chlamydia can cause a condition called nongonoccal urethritis (NGU), an infection of the urethra; and Epididymistis, which is inflammation of the epididymis where sperm are stored and matured.

Other prevalent STDs include gonorrhea and syphilis, which are also caused by bacterium in bodily fluids and transmitted through sexual intercourse. Gonorrhea also causes PID and infertility. Syphilis, on the other hand, causes psychological disorders and blindness if left untreated. It is important that you don't leave it untreated. Syphilis can be treated if caught in the early stages.

Human Immunodeficiency Virus (HIV) is another increasingly common STD. It is the virus that causes Acquired Immunodeficiency Syndrome (AIDS) and is very dangerous and even life threatening. It spreads primarily through sexual intercourse, blood transfusions, and sharing needles, but it is also transferable through breast milk. Therefore, being tested for HIV—both you and your partner—is critical before having your baby.

Genital Human Papillomavirus (HPV) is another common sexually transmitted disease. It is passed on through genital contact, most often during vaginal and anal sex. HPV may also be passed on during oral sex and genital-to-genital contact. HPV can be passed on between straight and same-sex partners—even when the infected partner has no signs or symptoms.

There are more than 40 types of HPV that can infect the genital area in both males and females. These HPV types can also infect the mouth and throat. Most people who become infected with HPV do not know they have it. It often leads to cervical cancer, which usually does not have symptoms until it is quite advanced.

Most people with HPV do not develop symptoms or health problems from it. In 90 percent of cases, the body's immune system clears HPV naturally within two years. Yet sometimes HPV infections persist and can cause genital warts, cervical cancer and other less common cancers of the vulva, vagina, penis, anus and oropharynx (back of the throat). For this reason, it is important for women to get regular screening for cervical cancer. Screening tests can find early signs of disease so that problems can be treated before they ever turn into cancer.

Vaccines can protect males and females against some of the most common types of HPV that can lead to disease and cancer. These vaccines are given in three shots. It is important to get all three doses to get the best protection. The vaccines are most effective when given at 11 or 12 years of age.

There are two vaccines for women and girls, called Cervarix and Gardasil, to protect females against the types of HPV that cause most cervical cancers.

Gardasil Background

On June 8, 2006, the FDA approved Gardasil for use in girls and women through the age of 26 years old. This vaccine prevents infection with the types of HPV that cause cervical cancer and genital warts. CDC's Advisory Committee on Immunization Practices (ACIP) recommends a routine three-dose vaccination of girls between the ages of 11 and 12. The vaccine is also recommended for girls and women of the age of 13 to 26 years who have not been vaccinated or has not received the three-dose.

Gardasil was tested in over 11,000 patients in the U.S. and around the world and found to be safe and effective in preventing serious HPV related diseases. These studies show that women who have never been infected by HPV types 6,11,16, or 18, the vaccine was highly effective in preventing precancerous lesions that often develop into cervical cancer, vaginal, vulva and preventing genital warts which is often caused by these HPV types.

This vaccine is an important tool in preventing cervical cancer in women all over the world. Every year 12,000 women are diagnosed with cervical cancer and almost 4,000 die from the disease in the US. Worldwide, cervical cancer is the second most common cancer in women, causing an estimated 470,000 new cases and 233,000 deaths per year.

Gardasil also protects against most genital warts and has also been shown to protect against anal, vaginal and vulvar cancers. Either vaccine is recommended for 11 and 12 year-old girls, and for females 13 through 26 years of age, who did not get any or all of the shots when they were younger. These vaccines can also be given to girls beginning at nine years of age. It is recommended to get the same vaccine brand for all three doses, whenever possible, so they can build up antibodies before they become sexually active.

One available vaccine (Gardasil) protects males against most genital warts and anal cancers. This vaccine is available for boys and men, nine through 26 years of age.[68]

Vaccine Monitors Safety

The FDA and CDC monitor the safety for all vaccines through the Vaccine Adverse Event Reporting Systems (VAERS). VAERS receives unconfirmed reports of possible side affects following the use of Gardasil and all vaccines licensed in the Unites States.

These reports are reviewed on a regular basis for any trends and concerns of possible side effects. All vaccines are produced in batches called lots and these lots are tested thoroughly and have to pass very high manufactured standards before they are put in use. The FDA studies each lot for any adverse effects associated with any lots to look for any unusual patterns. The FDA has seen no such patterns in the lots of Gardasil since the vaccine has been licensed.

In addition to VAERS, the CDC has two other systems in place to monitor safety of all licensed vaccines. The Vaccine Safety Datalink (VSD) Project works in a collaborative effort with the CDC and eight managed care organizations that monitors vaccine safety and immunization. The Clinical Immunization Safety Assessment (CISA) Network also works collaboratively with six academic centers in the United States to conduct research on vaccine associated adverse side effects.[69] (Please read end note 69 for an update on the vaccination Gardasil)

Genital warts usually appear as a small bump or group of bumps in the genital area. They can be small or large, raised or flat, or shaped like a cauliflower. HPV can cause normal cells on infected skin to turn abnormal. Most of the time, you cannot see or feel these cell changes. Genital warts can show up weeks after getting HPV. Cancer can show up years later.

Approximately 20 million Americans are currently infected with HPV. Another six million people become newly infected each year. HPV is so common that at least 50 percent of sexually active men and women get it at some point in their lives.

Other STDs and related infections include Genital Herpes, Hepatitis B, and Trichomoniasis. Herpes is transmitted sexual contact and can cause itching and burning of the genitals and anus. Sharing needles and sexual contact transmits Hepatitis B. This can cause nausea, vomiting, fever, loss of appetite, abdominal pain and liver damage. Trichomoniasis is a one-celled protozoan, a tiny parasite that travels between people during sexual intercourse. The incubation period between exposure and infection can range from five to 28 days. In women it causes foul-smelling vaginal discharge, genital itching and painful urination. Men who have trichomoniasis typically have no symptoms. Pregnant women who have trichomoniasis are at higher risk of delivering premature.[70]

If you have (or think you have) a sexually transmitted disease, discuss this with your specialist. Remember, too, that it is equally important to have your partner tested. If you do get pregnant while carrying a STD, you need to inform your OB-GYN. Herpes, for example, stays in your system forever and if the sores reappear while you are pregnant, your doctor may instruct you to have a C-section delivery instead of a vaginal delivery, since the baby could contract the herpes by passing through the vaginal canal.

It is daunting to realize that so many young people are having sexual relations and not using protection. As it is, we in the medical community are seeing a high incidence of chlamydia. If young people are not using protection, inevitably we will see more and more HIV. When young people experiment with sex they usually are not thinking of their future and their family's future, even though they are able to conceive and could very well do so. I gave a presentation to a group of high school students on STDs and the title was "Think of the Future not of the Moment." The sooner all sexually active partners understand this, the healthier they will be.

Chapter 12
Male Testing &
the Causes of Male Infertility

The evaluation of the male begins with a history, physical examination, and two semen analyses. Depending on where you receive your care, your specialist may have the male examined by the urologist as a routine infertility examination. Or you may see an urologist when your history or semen analysis raises a question about infertility.

Common Questions

Questions about male infertility and preparation for collecting semen specimens typically arise.

Does using a hot tub affect my fertility?

Sperm is very temperature sensitive and excessive heat can effect sperm production. It does not cause permanent damage but a hot tub should be avoided if you are going to give a semen specimen for an analysis. If you are in the hot tub on a continual basis (as opposed to being in one during a vacation), there is a good chance this could affect your fertility. The testes are on the outside of the body for a reason: a lower temperature environment is needed to produce healthy sperm. Sperm are reproduced every 72 days, so avoiding hot tubs for that period of time should enable sperm production to return to normal. Plan your vacation around the test!

Does it matter what kind of underwear I wear?

Another common question is whether or not it matters what kind of underwear a man wears. The old wives' tale that tight underwear causes decreased fertility has some basis in the truth, if negligibly. The excess heat applied to the testicles can decrease sperm production. However, the type of increased heat produced by tight clothing and/or underclothing has not been shown to elevate scrotal temperature. Hence, tight underwear has not been shown scientifically to cause increase in testicular heat and is not thought to have any effect on sperm production. Nevertheless, if you would like to try a change in clothing to see what happens, there is really no reason not to.

What is involved with the collection of a semen specimen and is it embarrassing?

The collection of a semen specimen is not easy for some men and it sometimes can be embarrassing for the patient. Everyone who works in any infertility program, including physicians, nurses and lab technicians are well acquainted with struggles and misgivings about this and truly understand the subtle heroics it takes for a man to produce and/or drop off a semen specimen. The generational contrast is humorous: strapping young men come running down the hall with the specimen cup in their hands with nothing to hide, while older men (maybe in their 40s and 50s) hide the specimen and avoid talking to anyone about why they are there. Don't be nervous.

I had a patient in his late 40s or early 50s who was very skittish. This first time he came to give me the specimen, he did not speak to me. He had only a note from his wife explaining what he was doing there. (If your wife tells you to go to the clinic to drop off a specimen, make sure you know what test you will be having that day.) I have often had male patients who would show up having no idea what test they were having done. They knew only that they were told by their partner to drop off a specimen. The lab performs several different tests on semen and needs to be sure that the correct test gets done. You should normally have a lab order from the specialist, but that doesn't always happen.

Some clinics may require you to book a semen analysis ahead of time so they know who to expect that day and for which test. Yet others don't require a booking so the lab has no idea how many patients could be showing up or what test is needed. (The tests will be explained in more detail later.) Thus, it is beneficial if you become familiar with the terms associated with sperm testing: determine ahead of time if you are there for an Intrauterine Insemination (IUI), a semen analysis, or sperm banking. It is very important that you talk to your partner and be aware of what test you are undergoing. In fact, everyone involved needs to be in the loop and understand clearly what is going on: you, your partner, your doctor and all medical staff in between. It makes it easier on everyone, but especially the male partner if he knows the procedure for which he is dropping off the specimen.

Let's go back to my friend who didn't want to talk to me when he dropped off his specimen. Time went on and he and his partner were undergoing IUIs so he came in more often to produce his specimen. In time he began talking to me and gained trust. Everyone felt more comfortable. We were even able to laugh together, despite the strain of the circumstances. In my lab patients could and would ask me anything. I guess I had the type of face that anyone could talk to. No question he asked was ever deemed silly. And as I have mentioned, this job has shown me how wonderful and sensitive men can be.

What Are Sperm, Anyway?

These little guys are very important, as you know. I mentioned earlier that they are very sensitive to high or low temperatures. So when you have finished collecting a specimen, don't put the cup in the refrigerator or place it near a hot stove or near the heater of your car in the winter when you are delivering the specimen to the lab. You'll kill them!

Did you ever wonder why the testes in man are located on the outside of the body as opposed to the inside? The reason is temperature. The production of healthy sperm requires a slightly lower temperature than core body temperature. If you are running a fever when you are scheduled to undergo a semen analysis test, reschedule. Allow enough time for the body temperature return to normal. An elevated body temperature will affect the sperm motility. Check with your RE, but you might even want to wait about two and a half months before giving a semen specimen after having had a fever. This is about the time it takes for sperm to develop from their immature stage to mature stage, which is about 72 days. So it's like getting a whole batch of new sperm. It's possible that you could be running a low-grade fever and not realizing it. If the sperm count is on the low side the specialist will ask for another specimen to be taken since this could be the reason why.

If you are collecting from home but delivering a specimen to a medical center you need to keep the specimen at body temperature. Time is critical. You should get the specimen to the lab within 45 minutes from the time of collection – and don't get a speeding ticket! You should be ready to leave the house before you collect and then place the specimen cup down the top of your pants, or inside your shirt tucked against your stomach. The sperm must be kept at body temperature.

If the female partner is delivering the specimen (for instance, if the male has to go to work), the same rules apply. She should be ready to go immediately following the collection. If she needs to get the children ready for the ride, she should wrap the specimen in the blanket of the bed until she is ready to leave. Then, en route, she should put the specimen cup down her bra (a very good place to hold the cup), or down the top of her pants. On top of everything else, she must not forget to bring some identification. All patients undergoing an IUI will be asked to show a picture ID. Most centers want the male present for an IUI drop off, but the female partner may be able to drop of a semen analysis with the proper identification.

The Semen Analysis Test

When you go to the lab to drop off a specimen or collect a specimen for a semen analysis, the lab technician will greet you and you will complete the necessary paper work for the test.

Semen analysis is a diagnostic test that tells the specialist the patient's sperm count, sperm motility, volume, pH (acidity: low pH or alkalinity: high pH), and sperm morphology (defined below). The male reproduces new sperm every 72 days and the sperm are at different stages of growth or maturity. So when the medical technologist looks at a specimen under the microscope there will be immature sperm, mature motile sperm, and non-motile sperm. Also, because millions are reproduced, there will be some abnormal shaped sperm. When the lab performs morphology, they are looking for normal shaped sperm. The semen analysis is a quick test with results being completed on the same day. This will help the specialist locate the problem area resulting in the infertility. The results are usually discussed on the second consult. If for any reason the specialist wants to repeat the test, it is nothing to worry about. Most specialists typically ask for two semen analysis tests because they can show different results.

On the day of your first consult the nurse will give you an instruction sheet for the semen analysis. This explains everything and may direct you to call the lab to book the appointment. Or the sheet may indicate specific hours during which you can show up for the test. In any case, be sure to read the instructions carefully. Most of the time these tests are done in the morning and during the week. (Even so, keep in mind that every center follows its own protocol.) Some centers may want you to collect your specimen on site at the center. Or they may allow you collect at home if you can deliver the specimen within 45 minutes from the time of collection.

Collecting a Specimen

Some patients look upon the occasion of semen collection on site with sheer terror. They are wondering what "the dreaded room" is like and if people can hear. I think every man who comes to the lab to give a specimen is looking around and wondering: Where is it? They may also be thinking, Where is that nurse? She probably has no personality, like on TV, when she gives you a magazine and shows you a bathroom. I sincerely believe the most dreaded aspect of collecting is the psychological confusion ahead of time.

Most collection rooms are approximately the size of a medium bathroom and include a sink and toilet. They provide magazines and some movies if a man feels it necessary, (hence the DVD player). Some patients bring in their own magazines.[71] Others don't need any visual accoutrements at all. It takes approximately 15 to 20 minutes for most men to collect a specimen. Your partner can join you in the collection room and help with your arousal, but the entire specimen needs to be collected.

The best way to collect the specimen is by masturbation. You should not collect the specimen by coitus interruptus, which is having intercourse with your partner and then withdrawing right before you ejaculate. There are two parts to the ejaculation, the first part containing the highest number of sperm. There is a good chance, if you attempt the collection by means of coitus interruptus, that the first part of the ejaculate will be lost. In addition, no lubricants should be used when collecting specimen.

This can be an easy process for some, but not so much for others. During your original consult, the center may have given you a set of instructions and a sterile specimen cup. The size of the cup should be one in which the opening is large enough to help in the collection of the complete specimen. Do not worry you are not to fill the cup. A typical volume for a single ejaculate is 2.5 ml to 5.0 ml. The cup can hold up to 120 mls.[72]

When the semen is ejaculated in the cup, it will be thick and may be covering only one area of the cup. Then with the passage of about 20 minutes, the specimen goes to a liquid consistency, which will normally fill the bottom of the cup.

When you are finished collecting the specimen you bring the cup to the lab technician, tucking it under your shirt if you are concerned that other patients may be in the area. The lab tech will ask if you lost any during collection and then will document the time of collection.

Some men have trouble producing a specimen on demand. This condition is called performance anxiety and a fair amount of patients have this condition. If you are collecting in the collection room and are unable to get a specimen, don't worry. Talk with someone in the lab and maybe try another day. Or maybe you would be more comfortable collecting from home. If that is the case, you would have to meet the time frame required to get the collection to the lab within 45 minutes. I cannot stress enough that this kind of thing happens all the time and you aren't alone. As a couple going through the program it is important that both partners understand the other's feelings and anxieties. The specialist may suggest sperm banking for a male patient with performance anxiety because once the female partner begins her cycle, a specimen must be produced at the right time. When you "sperm bank" an ejaculate, it will enable the male to be more at ease, knowing that there is always the safety net of the frozen backup.

Some men, for religious reasons or ethnic protocol will not masturbate. In this case the lab has special condoms, called Male Factor Pak, which do not contain lubricants or spermicides and is usable as a collection device when the couple has intercourse. The condom fits tightly and only comes in one size. The lab will review how to use it. If you have intercourse with this condom you will then have to be careful so as not to break it, in which case the specimen would be lost. Moreover, the condom may not cover the length of the penis so you will need to be careful that it does not get removed inside the female (this has happened). It is important to remember that it is a collecting device. It is the only device allowable if a couple has chosen intercourse as the means of collection.

The condom likewise can be used if the male is having trouble getting the specimen into the cup. Once finished remove the condom carefully and twist the plastic tie around the top of the condom so the specimen stays in the condom. Then place it in a cup.

The lab will ask you how many days abstinence have passed since your last ejaculation. In other words, they want to know how many days have passed between the time of the specimen collection and the last time you ejaculated. If you know a specimen collection is upcoming, you should avoid any sexual activity for at least two and four days to ensure that the sperm count will be at its highest number. For example, if you had ejaculated only a day before the scheduled collection, wait an additional full day (totaling two days) before the test. You have to give your body time to build up the volume and the sperm count again. On the other hand, if you have too many days abstinence from the last time you ejaculated, the semen analysis will register a higher count of less active sperm. Sperm are constantly going through a maturing stage and dying off. Too many days abstinence will show an increased number of non-motile sperm, which in turn, renders a low percentage of motile sperm.

A semen analysis measures the amount of semen produced and determines the number and quality of sperm. The normal ranges listed below after each category are from the World Health Organization (WHO)[73]. The semen analysis includes the following tests:

- *Total volume of the ejaculate:* Measuring the volume of the semen is important because a low volume could mean the patient may have a blockage in the male reproductive tract. Semen is the fluid that is produced by the male reproductive organs which supplies nourishment for the sperm and forms a medium for which they can swim. The lab will ask if any specimen was lost during collection and this will be noted on the report. This specimen is a fresh specimen collected in a sterile glass or plastic specimen cup and needs to be analyzed within one hour from the time of collection. (Normal volume is 2.5 to 5.0 ml.)

- *Total sperm count:* When the lab performs a sperm count they are counting motile sperm and non-motile sperm. Sperm are reproduced every 64 to 72 days, so there are many sperm in different stages of growth, from immature to mature sperm, in a single specimen. The lab refers to sperm that are not moving as non-motile. (Normal range is 20 million/ml or more). Oligospermia is the term used for low sperm count and Azoospermia is the term used when there is a complete absence of sperm in the ejaculate.
- *pH:* The pH is measured to see if the semen is alkaline or acid. (Normal pH for semen is alkaline eight to nine.)
- *Percent motility:* This is the percent of motile (moving) sperm out of the total number of sperm. (Normal range is greater than or equal to 50 percent motile sperm.)

143

- *Quality of motility:* This measures how the sperm are moving. Are they moving fast and with forward progression? Or does it look like the sperm are chasing its tail going around in a circle or moving like a snake? In normal circumstances the sperm needs to get to the egg, so it is optimal if they are moving fast and straight. (Remember from your first science class that it takes only one sperm to fertilize an egg.) Sperm motility is graded overall in a plus system. (1+ means it is barely moving; 2+ moving not with forward progression; 3+ and 4+ are considered normal, where the sperm are moving fast and in a forward progression.)

- *Sperm morphology:* This test involves the technician making a slide with a small bit of semen and stains the slide to look at each individual sperm. This enables the technician to grade the sperm as normal or abnormal according to the size and shape. Men produce millions of sperm so it is not unusual to have some that are abnormally shaped. A normal sperm has an oval head, neck and long straight tail. Abnormal sperm show head and/or tail defects. For example some sperm possess double heads or double tails, small heads, or large heads. The result is determined by the percentage of normal sperm counted. A percentage greater than or equal to 14 normal sperm cells is considered acceptable according to the strict criteria.

Retrograde Semen Analysis

There is a condition in some men called retrograde ejaculation. Normally when the semen is ejaculated it exits through the urethra and out the penis. In the case of retrograde ejaculation the semen is redirected into the bladder. There is a sphincter valve in the bladder, which closes so that the semen has only one way to go: out the urethra. Since the genital and urinary tracts are very close together (hence the term urogenital system) some men may have had to have surgery when they were young, related to the urinary system that over time can disrupt normal functioning. In this case a patient may say that when he ejaculates there is very little semen, if any. If the same patient were to urinate immediately following ejaculation he would see that the urine is cloudy indicating the semen (and sperm) in the urine. If you feel that you might fall into this category, mention this to your RE in the consult. He will order a retrograde semen analysis, which has its own special procedure for collection.

The two fluids, semen and urine, have opposite pH environments. The acid pH of the urine will not support sperm and keep them alive. Sperm require the basic pH (non-acidic) environment to live. This test requires neutralizing the acidic pH of the urine to a basic one. To accomplish this, the patient takes sodium bicarbonate, which is the chemical in Alka-Seltzer tablets.

In our clinic, the patient takes two Alka-Seltzer tablets in a large glass of water before going to bed on the night before test. Then he takes another two tablets with water in the morning within an hour before coming to the lab to collect the specimen. This will change the pH level in the urine enabling the sperm to survive.

The patient has to come to the lab for this test because time is of the essence. He will be given two specimen cups, one for ejaculation and one for urination, in that order. The urine specimen will be examined promptly. The lab analyzes the urine, checking for sperm, and will also do a subsequent semen analysis of the semen specimen. If the patient registers retrograde semen, sperm will be found in the urine sample and (assuming the pH is alkaline) will be moving. This sperm can be collected and used for insemination. I've seen this quite a few times and have done IUIs on these types of samples. The lab has a procedure that enables them to work fast to extract the sperm from the urine and use it for IUI or IVF procedures.

When semen analysis results are below normal values, the specialist will ask for a second specimen. The results can vary from one specimen to another. A male's results can be slightly off from the normal ranges and still can achieve pregnancy. Several factors can cause a low sperm count or no sperm.[74]

Other Male-Factor Issues

The specialist will review the results with the male partner. If it is determined that a male-factor infertility[75] is involved the specialist will recommend an urologist. The urologist will give you a complete physical examine and blood work. The male factor can include any disorder that affects the production or maturing of the sperm. This can include a low number of sperm, abnormally shaped sperm, low motility or no sperm at all. Male factor accounts for 40 percent of infertility cases.

If the results of the semen analysis read "No sperm seen," the specialist will ask for another specimen. Don't panic yet.

If you look at the male reproductive system, the sperm are made in the testicles and matured in the epididymis. When the male is sexually aroused and ejaculation occurs, the sperm and seminal fluid exits by means of a set of tubes called vas deferens and then the penis.

Some men have a condition in which they are missing the vas deferens. So when they ejaculate there is fluid but no sperm. It is possible for a Testicular Sperm Extraction (TESE) or Percutaneous Epididymal Sperm Aspiration (PESA) to be performed. This involves the sperm being taken out of the tissue and then used for IVF procedures. This will be mentioned in more detail in the Urology section.

In some semen analysis we'll see sperm that are bound together, called agglutination. Sperm can be stuck together by their tails, or by their heads or by both tails and heads. They can be moving as a group or look like they are struggling to pull apart from another. A possible cause of this is Antisperm antibodies.

Antisperm Antibodies

Our bodies develop antibodies to help protect our immune system against illnesses. Sometimes our bodies develop antibodies that attack the wrong thing, which can cause negative response. About 10 percent of infertile men will be diagnosed with having Antisperm antibodies, a condition that can significantly decrease chances of pregnancy.

In a normal situation the testes contain a natural barrier, known as the blood-testes barrier. This barrier acts a protective layer that prevents immune cells from being able to access sperm within the male reproductive tract. This barrier can be broken through injury to the testicles; undescended testes; twisted testes; and cancer. Absence of the vas deferens, a varicocele, or an infection can cause the immune cells to come into contact with the sperm. The sperm are considered a foreign body (antigen) to the immune cells and the immune cells produces antibodies against the sperm. These antibodies attach themselves to different areas on the sperm, which causes the sperm to stick together resulting in immobilization and prevent them from reaching the egg. A high percentage of men who have had a vasectomy reversal are more apt to have antisperm antibodies.[76]

Woman can also develop Antisperm antibodies in her cervical mucus, which further hinders fertility. Perhaps you have heard about the phenomenon of there being something in women that kills the sperm. This would be the cervical mucus. The cervix produces very thick mucus so no invading organisms or foreign particles can enter cervix or uterus. This protects the female reproductive tract. During ovulation the mucus thins out and allows sperm to pass through. But in some women—five to 10 percent—the mucus stays thick or may contain antibodies, which damage the sperm to the point that it may not make it to the egg. If a sperm does manage to reach the egg, the head is covered with antibodies and will not be able to fertilize the egg. In the past there was a test performed called the post coital test, which examined the mucus after intercourse to see if sperm are present. If they are present, but not motile, this may suggest there is something wrong with the mucus. Now with Assisted Reproductive techniques few physicians find benefit in testing sperm antibodies or cervical mucus as IUI and IVF both bypass this problem and seem to be the most helpful in treatment. An IUI can help the patient, either male or female, with anti-sperm antibodies. The lab will do a sperm wash, which helps break up the agglutinated sperm. This procedure detours the cervix and mucus and the washed sperm is placed directly into the uterus. In speaking with a RE from Georgia he did mention that abnormal cervical mucus is most often related to the use of clomiphene (Clomid). Many REs suggest IUIs if Clomid is part of the treatment regimen. However, in some cases, it may be necessary to incorporate IVF or ICSI into the treatment as well.[77]

Keep in Mind

As I said earlier, men are wonderful sensitive human beings and when there is a problem with their sperm count, it can come to them as quite a blow. Sometimes a patient will ask me: How is my sperm count after a washed specimen? Normally I would refer him to his nurse or RE for results, since they can explain in more detail. Yet, once in a while, I would be able to tell them the count was great, and you can see their big smile. In fact I'm sure I see their chests puff out a bit.

It is important to remember that the sperm count has no reflection on your libido or sex drive. The testes have two compartments, one with tubules that produce the sperm and one that is tissue between the tubules. This is where the Leydig cells are located, which produces the male sex hormone testosterone, which causes the sex drive. The tubules can be easily damaged but the Leydig cells are much more resistant to damage and will continually work in patients with testicular failure. So this is why a low sperm count can be such a surprise and a blow to one's sense of manhood. It is not associated with any other signs or symptoms.

Men take the news much differently. Many share common feelings of anger toward the wife or specialist. Perhaps they feel resentment because they feel having a baby is the women's job and resent their need to come to a fertility specialist. Many men have low self-esteem and experience a temporary setback in the desire for sex. They often feel guilty because the medical problem lies with them and that they are depriving their wives of the experience of motherhood. Male-factor infertility accounts for 40 to 50 percent of infertility diagnoses. Even so, there is help in dealing with this setback. Licensed social workers can help you both as a couple as you contend with your infertility diagnosis. The urge for fatherhood can be biologically as strong as the urge for motherhood. You are in this together as a couple. It is very important that you seek help as a couple and don't cast blame upon one or the other.[78]

Remember, no samples on or in:

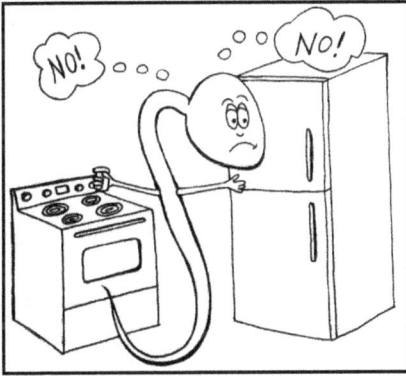

Chapter 13
Off to the Urologist

In the course of your infertility consultation as a couple, if it comes to light that the medical history of the male partner shows an abnormal semen analysis, the specialist refers him to a Urologist for further testing. An Urologist is a physician that specializes in the urinary tract for females and male and also specializes in the male reproductive tract.

Any testing already performed by the infertility specialist will be sent to the urologist. The urologist will scrutinize medical history and perform a complete physical exam. The urologists may run some or all of these tests:

- Checking the male reproductive organs: the size of the testicles and pubic hair
- Prostate exam
- Gynecomastia (the abnormal development of large mammary glands in males resulting in breast enlargement, which has generally been attributed to an imbalance of sex hormones or the tissue responsiveness to them)
- Complete blood work up (white and red blood cell counts)
- Complete Endocrine workup (hormone testing-

testosterone, LH Prolactin FSH and TSH)
- Ultrasound of the testicles (to check for tumors the physician can't feel or palpate.)

Genetic Testing includes:
- Cystic Fibrosis Blood test
- Karyotype (Blood work that shows a mapping of all the chromosomes in the body): men < 5 million sperm and Y chromosome deletion. Men carry the Y chromosome. Missing gene(s) on Y chromosome can cause Infertility, which could be a low, or no sperm count.
- Sperm DNA testing; specifically the DNA Fragmentation Index (DFI)
- Semen specimen

The Causes of Male Infertility

Men who live a healthy lifestyle are more likely to produce healthy sperm. The testes are responsible for sperm production (spermatogenesis). Normal production of sperm needs hormones and a healthy physical environment.

A wide array of treatment options are available for the many causes of male infertility. Sometimes male fertility can be improved by making simple lifestyle changes, such as abstaining from alcohol, tobacco, and illicit drugs. A healthy diet, sufficient exercise and proper amounts of vitamin B12, Vitamin C, selenium, folic acid and zinc also improve fertility.

In other instances physical and/or genetic problems

and injuries can affect the sperm production particularly if they occur at birth or a very young age during the growth of the reproductive system. These causes are related to problems with the testicles, sperm transportation, hormonal imbalances or ejaculatory issues. The following are conditions some young boys may encounter as infants while their reproductive systems are growing and maturing to young adults.

Undescended Testes[79]

Undescended testes are also known as Cryptorchidism. A baby's testicle should descend on its own within the first six to nine months of life. They start their descent down from the abdomen to the scrotum before birth. Once the testes have reached the scrotum, it is considered descended, even if it's pulled back (retracted) during an later examination. Some babies have a condition called retractable testes where the physician can't find them. There is a muscle flex that retracts the testes and the small testicle size before puberty. The testicles will completely drop during puberty. In this case surgery is not needed.

If the testicles have not descended by one year of age of the child, he should be evaluated and if necessary undergo surgery to reposition the testicle into the scrotum. This treatment is necessary because the higher body temperature may inhibit the normal development of the testicle, which would affect sperm production and cause infertility. Further, the chance that the undescended testicle could form a tumor increases, as well as the chances for injury or testicular torsion (twisting). Boys with an empty scrotum also have a better chance of inguinal hernias, not to mention potentially causing a child to be embarrassed.

Cryptorchidism is the most common genital abnormality in boys, affecting approximately 30 percent of baby boys born prematurely and about four percent born at term. In about half the babies the testes will descend on their own by six months. If this doesn't happen it is important to seek treatment as soon as possible since undescended testicles may be damaged.

Varicocele

A varicocele is a single or mass of varicose veins in the scrotum. They seem to occur in adolescence years when the testes are growing and when there is a larger blood supply for oxygen and nutrients to the area. If the valves aren't functioning properly and the veins can't handle the extra blood, it begins to pool in the scrotum. Varicoceles may cause damage to the testes by inhibiting proper growth. One teste may be smaller than the other and this one will produce less sperm.

A varicocele affects the sperm because the large amount of blood present increases the overall temperature, which affects or kills the sperm and can also cause abnormal sperm morphology. It is usually found only in one testicle and often in the left side. Depending on its size it can be painful. A physician can usually palpate (feel with his hand) a varicocele or it can be diagnosed by means of an ultrasound. Men may father a child initially, but as time goes on will have secondary infertility, trouble having a second child.

The common treatment method for this condition is called microsurgery (microsurgical ligation), which ties off the defective veins. Another type of surgery, called percutaneous embolism, blocks the veins. Repair to a varicoceles can improve the sperm count but it is controversial whether the actual repair can cause pregnancy. In some patients varicoceles cause low sperm counts and depending how low the count is surgery may not improve the count. The RE's plan could be IVF for the couple and, if this is the case, the male may not have the surgery for the varicocele.[80]

Testicular Injury or Torsion

Sports injuries can cause injury to the testes or torsion. That is why it is very important for young boys to wear an athletic supporter at any time when there is an activity that could lead to a groin injury. Testicular injuries can be very serious and cause bruising, internal bleeding to one or both of the testes.[81]

If the spermatic cord becomes twisted (torsion), this is considered a medical emergency. When testicular torsion occurs the blood flow is cut off to the teste and surrounding tissue and can cause the tissue to die. This area could become infected and the teste may have to be removed. Any time there is trauma to the testes it can affect sperm production. You may have heard of gastric torsion, which occurs frequently in horses and large breed dogs (such as a Great Dane). If they get running or playing too hard their stomach flips over and cuts off all the blood flow to the stomach and intestines. If surgery is not done as soon as possible, the dog will die.

Mumps

Mumps is a virus that affects the salivary glands and in some cases can affect one or more of the testes causing inflammation called Orchitis. The scrotum area will be sore and swollen. This inflammation can cause shrinkage of the affected tissue in the testes and in severe cases can cause sterility. Mumps, like other viruses, seems to be cropping up more frequently, especially in young men in their late 20s. This disease is more severe when it affects adults. It is rare to cause complete infertility, though it may cause a low sperm count. Men are encouraged to get the mumps vaccination if they never contracted it as a child. If you don't know if you had the infection as a child your physician can draw your blood for an antibody titer to determine if you possess the antibodies for mumps. The vaccination known as the MMR (for mumps, measles and rubella) is usually given to children when they are two years of age.[82]

Congenital Absence of Vas Deferens (CAVD)

Congenital Absence of Vas Deferens is a condition in which a portion or all the male's reproductive ducts are missing.[83] The vas deferens carries the sperm from the testes to the penis and there are two one from each teste. CAVD causes obstruction of the sperm reproduced in the testes, since they have no way of getting out.

Some men are born with only one tube missing while others may have the condition in both. The condition can occur by itself or it may be a sign of Cystic Fibrosis. Many men with the absence of the vas deferens may not have any other signs of Cystic Fibrosis, but may have mild respiratory problems. Cystic Fibrosis is one of the more common genetic testing that is done with couples entering a program (please be aware of this and have the other partner tested if he happens to have CAVD).

Some STDs cause blockage in the epididymis or tubes, causing tubal scarring.

In any of these cases, sperm can be retrieved by sperm extraction, which bypass the blocked or damaged tubes. Once sperm is successfully retrieved an IVF cycle can be done. If a sufficient amount of sperm is retrieved then the sperm can be frozen for use in other cycles.[84]

Testicular Sperm Extraction (TESE) is a process by where a small portion of tissue is extracted that, hopefully, contains viable sperm usable for the IVF - ICSI cycle. Intracytoplasmic sperm injection (ICSI) means the sperm are injected directly into the egg. This type of extraction is done on men who are unable to produce sperm through ejaculation due to missing or damaged tubes. Their semen specimen would show visible no sperm (azoospermic). The TESE procedure and ICSI have diminished the need for donor sperm making it possible for the patient to father a child.

Percutaneous Epididymal Sperm Aspiration (PESA) is a process by which a needle is placed in the epididymis where sperm are stored and matured. Microsurgical Epididymal Sperm Aspiration or MESA is a delicate process by which sperm is aspirated using a microscope and taken from an area close to the tubal blockage.[85] These are done for patients with blocked tubes, followed by the ICSI.

I remember two separate couples with this condition. Their semen analysis reflected no visible sperm. The patients then had a sperm extraction or aspiration performed and both were able to do an IVF cycle. As a result, both couples gave birth to a set of twins on the first try.

Infections

Infections and diseases such as tuberculosis, influenza and STDs can cause testicular atrophy. STDs are the most common infection that causes infertility, including gonorrhea, chlamydia and syphilis. STDs cause infertility by blocking the tubes. In these infections a low sperm count or a low motility count is evident.

Dental abscesses also have been known to cause a low sperm count. Hormonal replacement can help some of these conditions, but surgery will be the treatment for blockages. Treat the STDs with antibiotics. Condoms should be used in the future to prevent further infections

Klinefelter's Syndrome

In the human body men have an XY chromosome and woman have an XX chromosome. In a certain genetic condition a male will have an extra X chromosome, so he would be XXY. This is called Klinefelter's Syndrome. This may be evident in pea-sized hard testicles and enlarged breasts. The physical traits of the syndrome become more evident during puberty. Since these boys do not produce as much testosterone, they often have a less muscular body, less facial and body hair, broader hips and enlarged breasts. XXY males in adulthood carry similar physical features as men without the condition, although they are often taller. Characteristics in adults vary widely and may include little or no signs other than a lanky build with some degree of increased breast tissue (gynecomastia). Affected males are often infertile or may have reduced fertility. IVF can be successful for some patients.

A blood test for chromosome analysis is used to confirm this diagnosis. If discovered in puberty the young person can be given testosterone to help the physical symptoms. However, the man will have either very little or no sperm production. Klinefelter's Syndrome may eventually cause all active testicular structures to atrophy. Once testicular failure has occurred, improving fertility is impossible. Some men don't realize they have this condition until they start trying to conceive a child and are unsuccessful.[86]

Retrograde Ejaculation

This condition, as mentioned earlier, causes the semen to be ejaculated into the bladder rather than out through the urethra because of the failure of the bladder sphincter to close during ejaculation. Evidence of the presence of this disorder can be seen in a low ejaculate volume (or none) and cloudy urine after ejaculation. The condition affects 1.5 percent of infertile men. It may be controlled by medications like decongestants, which contract the bladder sphincter, or surgical reconstruction of the bladder neck to restore normal ejaculation. In some cases young children get bladder neck surgery to help urine flow, though the surgery may cause a retrograde ejaculation later on. (The urinary tract and reproductive tact are so closely related that any surgery in this area can cause a retrograde.)

If the male partner has this condition the sperm can be removed from the urine for an IUI or IVF procedure. However, this must be done quickly to get the sperm out of the urine, change the pH from acid (urine) to basic pH so the sperm can survive. Once they are out then we can perform a regular sperm wash.

Hormonal Abnormalities

The testicles need pituitary hormones to be stimulated to make sperm. If these are absent or severely decreased, the testes cannot produce sperm to maximum capacity. It is important for men to understand that if they take androgens (steroids) for bodybuilding, either by mouth or injection, it shuts down the production of hormones for sperm production.

Hormonal Imbalances

If you're a male with infertility problems your medical team will do a hormonal profile. It is important to check this aspect of your body's functioning in order to rule out serious medical conditions; to get more information on the sperm-producing ability of the testes; and inform your medical team whether to go ahead with hormonal treatment.

Hormones run our bodies and when any one of them is imbalanced, it can wreak havoc in any of our bodily systems. The testes need pituitary hormones to be stimulated to make the sperm. There are three main hormones that play an important role in the male reproductive system. FSH (Follicle stimulating hormone) is needed for sperm reproduction and LH (luteinizing hormone) is needed for testosterone production. When a man has a low sperm count or low motility the urologist will have his blood drawn to test for those hormones.

The hypothalamus and pituitary system regulates the chain of events that enables the testes to produce sperm. A disruption or failure of the brain and or pituitary to produce these hormones will affect the sperm production. The pituitary gland can fail to produce enough LH and FSH to stimulate the testes and testosterone sperm production.

Other hormones that may disrupt male infertility include:

Hyperthyroidism, Hypothyroidism:
The thyroid gland controls many systems in our bodies. Either high or low levels of thyroid hormones affect sperm count and motility. Low levels of thyroid hormones could affect libido. Thyroid replacement therapy can help elevate sperm counts.

Congenital Adrenal Hyperplasia (CAH):

CAH refers to a group of genetic disorders of the adrenal gland. CAH can affect boys and girls. This condition means their bodies are lacking an enzyme needed by the adrenal glands to produce the hormones cortisol and aldosterone. Without these hormones the adrenal glands produce more androgens (male sex hormone). Symptoms can range from mild to serious. In some girls that are born with the serious case may show abnormal genitals before symptoms appear. Boys will severe cases will appear normal at birth. Some children with a mild case may not be diagnosed until late adolescence. Boys and girls with this condition will appear to be entering puberty early. Changes may include: early development of male characteristics, pubic hair or armpit hair, and well developed muscles and enlarged penis. Females with high androgens will have irregular menstrual cycles. Treatment includes taking hormone replacement therapy, which is usually taking cortisol on a daily basis.[87]

Hyperprolactinemia

Just as in women, males also produce prolactin. Increased levels of prolactin can have an adverse affect of the testicles and can cause decreased levels of testosterone. So typically these men may have decreased sperm count, decreased libido and erectile dysfunction. If a male patient has hyperprolactinemia, he may not show any physical signs, which could make diagnosing difficult. But some men may develop a condition called gynecomastia, which causes the breasts to become enlarged. This is often a sign of high levels of prolactin.

If diagnosed properly it can be treated with medications. If prolactin levels keep increasing, it could signal that there is a small benign tumor on the pituitary gland. (This would be diagnosed with blood tests and/or an MRI. The tumor is called a prolactinomas.) The goal of treatment is to lower the prolactin level to a normal level and to shrink the prolactinomas.

Most prolactinomas can be safely treated with medications that will shrink the tumor. Or, the tumor can be removed surgically. If there is a male factor most REs and urologists will include prolactin as part of the blood work for hormones. It doesn't hurt to ask the physician to have this checked.[88]

Testosterone

Testosterone is a hormone made by your body and is responsible for the normal growth and development of the male sex organs and for maintenance of other sexual characteristics. In men, testosterone is produced in the testes, the reproductive glands that also produce sperm. The amount of testosterone produced by the testes is regulated by the hypothalamus and the pituitary gland. Some effects of testosterone may include:

- Growth and maturation of prostate and other male sex organs
- Development of male hair distribution such as facial hair
- Changes in body muscle mass and strength and fat distribution

165

- Sex drive and sexual function
- Mood and energy level
- Bone strength

Normal Levels of Testosterone

In healthy men, normal testosterone levels (also known as T levels) fall between 300 ng/dL and 1200 ng/dL.[89] The brain and the testes work together to keep testosterone in this range. When levels of testosterone are below normal, the brain signals the testes to make more. When there is enough testosterone, the brain signals the testes to make less.

What is Low Testosterone? "Do you have low T"

As men age testosterone levels start to decline gradually. Nevertheless, some men can have a low testosterone that occurs when your body isn't producing normal levels of testosterone. This leads to a medical condition called hypogonadism.[90] Common symptoms include reduced sex drive, decreased energy, loss of body hair or reduced shaving, and depressed mood.

Much of the sexual dysfunction humans experience is related to low testosterone and lack of exercise. A dramatic drop in testosterone is followed by weight gain in men. Obesity is not only related to diabetes but also related to lower testosterone levels. This is because the aromatase enzyme in your body's fat cells transforms your testosterone into estradiol (E2), which is an active form of estrogen. High levels of E2 stimulate the sex hormone binding globulin (SHBG), which binds up the remaining testosterone. SHBG acts like a switch turning on and off the availability of testosterone. It is important to get testosterone, a free testosterone and SHBG hormone levels drawn to really show how much testosterone you have. Testosterone is in the blood and is bonded to molecules and "free testosterone" is free flowing in the blood, which gives you the libido.

Men go through their own type of menopause like women called andropause, which is a decline in testosterone. Testosterone is a major barometer for the aging process. Starting at the age of 40 men's testosterone generally declines at a rate of one percent each year. As a young male they enjoy the highest levels of testosterone from ages 21 to 24 years. By age 55 the testosterone level might be half of what they were when they were young.

Common effects of the onset of andropause as men age can be low libido, erectile dysfunction, night sweats and, yes, some can have hot flashes. Those who experience this feel as if it is affecting every aspect of their lives. This is because testosterone controls so many functions in the male's body. The good news is, your doctor can diagnose it easily and can begin hormonal replacement treatments based upon a medical history, exam, symptoms, and certain blood tests. Treatment for replacement therapy can be done with supplemental testosterone, which will actually slow down the aging process. Talk to your specialist or urologist about hormone replacement therapy. [91]

Do you have High T?

High testosterone levels in men may be caused by genetics, pituitary gland problems or from taking testosterone supplements or anabolic steroids. Some side effects of high testosterone levels are temporary and resolve when testosterone levels return to normal. Other effects may be permanent and require medical treatment. Men with high testosterone levels should have regular medical exams, including screenings for prostate cancer.

Infertility is a temporary side effect of high testosterone levels in men, due to reduced production of sperm and shrinking of the testicles.

Taking Illegal Steroids [92]

"Did you notice those guys with big muscles at the gym or on the beach? The muscles may be from 'just plain old fashioned hard work in the gym' or they could be from using anabolic steroids or performance enhancing drugs (PED). Those that use anabolic steroids or PEDs to build and repair muscle are doing damage to their testicles. These testosterone-based hormones are very bad for men who eventually want to have children. They actually work almost like a contraceptive. When a man is taking anabolic steroids, it is virtually impossible for him to get his partner pregnant."

How do anabolic steroids affect male fertility?

Sperm are produced in the body when the hormones luteinizing hormone (LH) and follicle-stimulating hormone (FSH) secreted by the brain and work directly on the testicles and the cells present in the testes called Leydig cells. The Leydig cells then in turn produce the major male hormone testosterone, which is needed for sperm production. When the cells produce testosterone it causes the testicles to have a very high level of testosterone, although there is a normal level in the blood stream. When men use anabolic steroids, they trick the body into thinking that the testicles DO NOT have to produce testosterone. When this happens, the amount of testosterone in the testicles is extremely low, despite normal or very high levels in the bloodstream. Because of this follicle stimulating hormone FSH is not produced and this combination causes the testicles to shrink and to produce little if any sperm.

The good news is sperm can come back after stopping steroid use, it could as little as 3 months or up to one or two years depending on the length of time the steroids were being used. Sometimes after a period of time from stopping the performance enhancing drugs, medical therapy can help the ability to start sperm production by giving the hormone human gonadotropin (hCG) and if that doesn't help then a form of FSH called human menopausal gonadotropin can be added to improve the chances to return the sperm. It is known that long-term use of steroids produces dangerous and long-lasting detrimental side effects, which may not be reversible. Some of these side effects include aggressive behavior, baldness, acne, prominent breasts, liver disease, high blood pressure, heart attack or stroke. In adolescents, it may result in stunted growth and accelerated puberty changes. PEDs can also cause sexually dysfunction and loss of sex drive.

I had a patient who was a body builder ask me how his sperm would be after stopping taking steroids for six months. I told him I wouldn't know until I looked under the microscope. But I also stressed the importance of quitting steroid use. Fortunately for him the sperm did comeback. The best advice is to never start taking PEDs if you are planning a family and you want to be healthy.

I attended a recent urology talk and the guest speaker was Dr. Stephen Lazarou from Newton Wellesley Hospital in Massachusetts. He said, "If you are pursuing fertility, taking any testosterone causes a negative feedback on the pituitary reducing LH and FSH release, which in turns causes testicular atrophy hence reduced spermatogenesis. Therefore men with a low testosterone, I would use Clomid to boost their endogenous testosterone production and maintain sperm production." A testosterone level in the high normal range is fine. However, a high FSH is typically suggestive of primary testicular failure."[93]

Your urologist can treat hormonal imbalances with medications. If an imbalance of hormones is the major reason for infertility the urologist or your RE will send you to an endocrinologist who specializes in the body's hormone secreting glands.

All the hormones mentioned—FSH, LH, Estrogen and Testosterone—are the same hormones in the female reproductive system. It is the amounts of these hormones that differ in males and females and have the different functions. The medication Clomid, mentioned above, is given to women to induce ovulation. But obviously it has a different affect on men. Hormone replacement can take up to four months before seeing any results.

Male Sexual Dysfunction

A sexual problem or sexual dysfunction refers to a problem in any phase of sexual arousal to intercourse that exists and can affect male fertility. Sexual dysfunction can be a physical or psychological problem and sometimes it is hard to tell the difference. I found a wonderful article on performance anxiety, written by Dr Stanley Ducharme, Ph.D. who is a sex therapist and works with couples and their relationships. He has graciously granted me permission to reprint the article here, since the main mission of this book is to help couples to understand exactly what is going on.

Understanding Performance Anxiety
by Stanley Ducharme, Ph.D. [94]

"Millions of men, regardless of age, relationship or orientation suffer from sexual performance anxiety. This condition in sexual situations occurs when a man anticipates some form of problem occurring during the sexual act. As a result of this anticipation, the man becomes anxious or panicked while attempting to be sexually active. This translates into problems with erections, premature and delayed ejaculation or a lack of desire to have sex.

Although performance anxiety can also occur with women, it is less understood and less common. Often it is called anorgasmia or the inability to have an orgasm. Sometimes, it is called vaginismus or the inability to relax the muscles of the vagina.

In this short paper however, our primary focus is on male performance anxiety since the term usually refers to a man's anxiety about his sexual performance. This anxiety can be deep routed. Many sex therapists believe that a man's anxiety about sex is related to his underlying fears and insecurities. Frequently, many of these feelings have never been verbalized.

Anxiety about sex can take many forms. Some men have fears about being rejected, disappointing a partner or becoming embarrassed about the quality of an erection. Other men have fears regarding their reputation or anxieties related to their masculinity or sexual orientation. In this area, feeling inadequate can be especially painful. Performance anxiety hits a man in his most vulnerable and insecure areas. It's different for each man.

Medications such as Viagra, Cialis or LaVitra are very effective for many men. Often, they are extremely helpful in restoring a man's confidence as well. They allow him to worry less about his erections and to focus on other areas of the sexual act. Sometimes however, even these medications don't completely remove the anxiety and a man's fears regarding his performance. These anxieties can be deeply rooted.

Having anxiety about sex is a difficult situation to reverse. Unfortunately, it is very common and can happen to anyone at any age and at any time. Sexual performance anxiety can start from a very brief simple event even in very stable, emotionally healthy individuals. Sometimes even a single time in which the man loses an erection can be enough to raise doubts and cause anxiety the next time. Although this happens to every man at certain occasions, it can begin a downward spiral causing problems of confidence in and out of the bedroom. The more frantic you become the worse the problem will become. This can be a very slippery slope!

Anxiety is intended by nature to be a warning system of a threat or danger. In such cases, your brain becomes alert, your muscles tense for running or battle and other parts of your body, such as digestion, shut down while you are in stand-by mode. In the sexual situation, if our warning system tells us that there may be a problem then we are more likely to have a problem. The warning system causes the problem. This is a self-fulfilling fear.

So, if a man's brain warns him that there may be a problem during sex, there will be a problem because of the warning. A man's warning system releases chemicals that interfere with his sexual performance. We were not made to be anxious and have sex at the same time.

Sex therapists use a technique called sensate

focus to help men with performance anxiety. This technique encourages a couple to remove all stress from the sexual act. Sensate focus was first used by Masters and Johnson and aims to get a man to stop thinking about erections and his performance. Instead, the goal of sensate focus exercises is to get the man to focus on the feelings and sensations of sexual arousal. Rather than thinking about performance, the goal is to experience each touch, sensation, smell, movement, sound and taste of the sexual act.

Men who are experiencing performance anxiety tends to perceive sex as an obligation or a job that needs to be accomplished. Performance anxiety diminishes sexual drive. As a result, men with performance anxiety often avoid sexual activity. For these men, sex is no longer fun and enjoyable because they have lost sight of the pleasures involved in sexual contact. Performance anxiety causes the man to focus on the mechanics of sex rather than the pleasure, sensations and excitement. They are thinking about sex rather than enjoying it. Sex is best when you can shut the mind off and stop thinking.

To accomplish this goal of getting a man to enjoy sex again, sex therapists try to take all the expectations and pressure away. They instruct the couple not to have intercourse and not to be concerned about the erection. This may be difficult and therapists realize that not everyone can ignore the erection and the goal of having intercourse. The idea is that if the couple can be together a number of times without the expectation and pressure of performing then the whole experience begins to take on a completely different flavor.

What is important during sex are the sensations that the couple experience; the ways they learn to pleasure each other; the sexual fantasies and the feelings of each becoming aroused. If a couple have difficulty not thinking about the mechanics of sex, the therapist might suggest that they keep their clothes on or wear their underwear for the first few times. Then, it really doesn't matter if the man's achieves an erection or not. Without the pressure, hopefully the man can begin to relax.

When the couple feels relaxed in this situation, the next step might be for them to communicate, caress and touch without clothes. The focus however is always on the pleasure and the enjoyment. Without worry about the erection or his performance, sex for the man is not a job that needs to be done. It can be a positive and pleasurable experience.

When the man's performance becomes less important he's not going to be thinking so much about it. He'll be experiencing other things like erotic sensations, sexual pleasure or the emotional closeness between the two people. Without the worries, most men will begin to actually enjoy the experience of sex, which will result in arousal. This is an example of reverse psychology! The less you care about your arousal the better it will be.

In summary, many men with sexual difficulties tend to over-think about their performance rather than staying in the moment and enjoying the sexual sensations and feelings. In the instant that you began to think about performance or worrying about how you are doing, you become an observer rather than a participant. At that time, the body's warning system becomes activated and your sexual arousal becomes diminished.

Performance anxiety is a common situation for most men at different times in their life. Changing how a person thinks and learning to forget about the quality of the sexual act is certainly easier said than done. The key to overcoming this problem however is in being completely honest with yourself. This mean really convincing yourself deep down inside that it is ok if your erection and performance are not perfect.

If you can convince yourself that sexual performance and erections are not essential then there is a much better chance that your body will become sexually aroused? Great sex is about not thinking. It is about letting yourself go and sinking into the experience of physical and emotional intimacy."

Performance anxiety can also affect a patient when, they are told to produce a specimen *right now,* for an ART procedure such as IUI or IVF. They might struggle to produce the specimen, and the anxiety may increase with the more pressure they feel. Do you have any idea what a man feels like in this situation?

If I had a patient who couldn't produce and lets say he came out of the collection room without a specimen. I would take them to the side and ask them if everything is okay. They usually say they couldn't produce, they didn't think it would be that difficult. I would explain to them that this happens frequently and if the lab allows maybe next time he could try to collect at home. If this seems to be a problem, I would mention sperm banking, where they can freeze specimens prior to procedures and if they can't collect the day of the procedure then the lab could use a frozen specimen. I think this gives male patients extra confidence and assurance that there will be a specimen for the procedure. A male patient is under tremendous pressure because, to this point, his partner has taken these medications for an IVF cycle and the day has come when he must deliver. It can be crushing for him not to be able to produce a specimen. I would give them the option if possible to try at home, though it is important to remember that there is a time limit for specimen to be returned within 45 minutes from time of collection. Men are so honest and shy, but at the same time, they felt comfortable talking to me. (Men: it is important that you feel comfortable with your medical team for this reason.)

The RE might speak to the couple about sperm banking. This means saving the sperm by freezing it if ejaculation occurs any time before the procedure and if, when the day came, the male could not produce. In this case, the lab can take a frozen vial and use that specimen for the procedure.

It helps the male partner to know he has a back up. It diminishes some of the pressure and may enable him to produce a fresh specimen as needed. If the patient decided to sperm bank, I would tell them simply to bring me a specimen any time on a particular day up till about noontime. Some of my patients would show up and be quite proud that they were able to produce. After a few times they didn't have an issue anymore. But it is advantageous to have a banked specimen, just in case.

There are other sexual dysfunctions that men can have and can be related to performance anxiety.

Erectile Disfunction (ED)

Erectile dysfunction is characterized by the inability to maintain an erection or sustain it long enough to achieve sexual intercourse. This can happen occasionally. But when it becomes a pattern, it may be time to see your doctor. This condition is also known as impotence and effects up to 30 million men in America. ED can be caused by mental or physical problems or a combination of both. Men who are depressed or have some emotional problems may have no interest in having sex. There may be also physical problems relating to the blood flow to the penis. During stimulation, the brain sends out signals for smooth muscles in the body to relax which sends the blood flowing throughout the body and flow down to the penis. The penis fills with blood and causes an erection.

Without proper blood flow there is a greater chance of having ED.

Some of these physical problems can include high blood pressure, high cholesterol and diabetes. Some medications have side effects that can cause ED, like blood pressure and antidepressants. ED can be treated. It is important to see a urologist and explore together all aspects of the situation. This condition affects a lot of men so don't feel shy about talking to your RE. They can prescribe medications that will help increase the blood flow.[95] Sometimes it can be caused by a hormonal imbalance that can be checked easily and treated with testosterone.[96]

Premature Ejaculation

When it comes to conceiving a child two things have to happen: vaginal penetration and ejaculation. Sometimes, however, ejaculation happens before penetration. This is when infertility may come into the picture. Occasional premature ejaculation is common in men. But if ejaculation before penetration occurs more than a few times, you will want to seek medical help. Any of the ART, IUI or IVF treatments can help patients with this condition.

Ejaculatory Incompetence

Delayed ejaculation or retarded ejaculation is the inability of a man to reach climax and ejaculate in the partner's vagina. He is able to ejaculate through foreplay or masturbation but not during intercourse. Problems of delayed ejaculation tend to be rare and not well understood by psychologists, medical doctors or urologists.

For this reason finding the right professional that has experience and realizes the seriousness of the problem can be a difficult process in itself.

Ejaculation problems can have a devastating affect on a man's self-esteem. He feels he has little to offer the relationship and communication between partners may become strained.

Reasons for this could stem from medications, increase use of alcohol or drugs, or could be the result of thoughts that can come from religious background that might suggest sex is wrong. It could also stem from sexual abuse in the past. This disorder causes considerable distress, anxiety and loss of sexual confidence.

Because of the lack of information regarding delayed ejaculation, the most successful approach for sex therapists is engaging both members of the couple in addressing the problem. Resolving the problem seems to work best when the couple can work as a team. If the man is in a relationship, he needs support and understanding from his partner.

Sex can serve as a trigger to bring back painful emotional feelings from the past. Ignoring these important emotional issues can lead to difficulties in resolving the problem.

Under the right circumstances and with ongoing motivation, ejaculation disorders can be overcome. The first step is deciding to seek treatment and finding the proper profession that has experience and understands.[97]

Conclusion

You have seen the urologist been examined and tested thoroughly. Hopefully, the urologist has identified any problems that might exist in the male factor. In some cases you may have had a surgical procedure like removing a varicocele, or you may have been put on hormonal treatment. In any case, at some point you will repeat a semen analysis test to see if there are changes. The urologist will tell you the proper time to have this done. He will communicate with your infertility specialist so that both doctors are on the same page with your treatment. You'll go back to the infertility specialist and have another consult to see what the new plan maybe for the two of you.

If you have any blocked ducts or missing the vas deferens, the urologists will perform the surgery for sperm extraction at the exact time the infertility specialist is performing the egg retrieval for IVF.

Chapter 14
Advanced Testing for Infertility

New studies and research are constantly being performed to develop and refine infertility treatments. Some hospitals have clinical trials in infertility treatments that are looking for male, female or couples, depending upon the research. Patients may be eligible to participate if they fill the requirements of the study and this may help with some infertility costs. As a patient staying up-to-date on infertility, research helps patients be better informed and thus, empowered. I wanted to share some recently new testing to help in the treatment of infertility.

For the Female:

There are two hormones in the female, AMH (Anti-Mullerian Hormone) and DHEA (Dehydroepiandrosterone) that aid in the diagnosis of DOR (Diminished Ovarian Reserve).

For the Male:

Recently, there has been increased emphasis on the evaluation of sperm quality. This is due, in part to the fact that a semen analysis by itself is of limited value. Sperm counts, for example, fluctuate significantly from day to day in most men. Researchers are looking at the quality and integrity of the sperm. The test is called DNA Fragmentation Index (DFI) and even more recent research has a new test in finding the "best sperm"

Some clinics may be testing these already and using the results to help them verify certain diagnosis. Keep in mind the tests may not be covered by insurance and can be very expensive.

What is Anti-Mullerian Hormone?

As a women ages, her supply of eggs gradually declines over time until the eggs are depleted at menopause. We expect the ovary to age in a certain way, but there are times when it doesn't behave as expected. This is why testing for ovarian reserve is a necessary part of the initial evaluation for infertility patients of any age. The term "ovarian reserve" refers to a women's current egg supply and is closely related to the reproductive potential. The greater number of remaining eggs, the better chances is for conceiving. Conversely, low ovarian reserve diminishes the chances for conceiving.

To measure ovarian reserve most specialists use the Day-3 and Day-10 FSH (CCT), which is the usual work up for a new fertility patient.

Every month, the pituitary gland sends out FSH to tell your ovaries to get to work growing and maturing the follicles that will hold and release an egg. The new indicator for ovarian reserve that some REs are testing for is the Anti-Mullerian Hormone (AMH). Cells that line the small ovarian follicles release this protein and there is a direct correlation between AMH levels and the number of pre-antral follicles and antral follicles (also called resting follicles or "good" follicles). AMH is measured in the small antral follicles. As the follicle matures AMH decreases. This is why AMH levels are thought to reflect the size of the remaining egg supply and gives an indication of the ovarian reserve and a women's fertility status. So knowing the AMH blood level in conjunction with the patient's age is useful in determining a reliable assessment of the ovarian reserve and how well a patient might respond to the injectable FSH drugs.

AMH can be used for:

1. Evaluating Fertility potential and ovarian response in IVF - Serum AMH levels correlate with the number of early antral follicles. This makes it useful for predicting your ovarian response in an IVF cycle. Women with low AMH levels are more likely to be poor ovarian responders.

2. Measuring Ovarian Aging - Diminished ovarian reserve is signaled by reduced baseline serum AMH concentrations. Women with poor ovarian reserve and who have poor ovarian response, have low levels of AMH.

3. AMH can verify a high Day-3 FSH or abnormal CCT

4. AMH is more stable and can be measured anytime during the cycle

5. Women older than 35 years old or women that have unexplained infertility

6. It is believed that women with PCOS have an elevated level of AMH, which would help in the diagnosis.

7. Women with an abnormal AMH level may want to confirm the need to move on to donor eggs for IVF.[98]

It is often the case that women who have been putting their careers before their family have difficulty getting pregnant when they are ready to have a family. It's only natural that women wonder if they are still ovulating and how much time they have left before their eggs run out. The AMH test claims to answer these questions. I would speak to your specialist about looking at the test in this manner, because it could be a very small window of time.

Whatever the use, fertility experts currently believe that the AMH test is about 70 percent accurate.[99]

In order to give a complete fertility assessment, AMH results need to be interpreted by a fertility specialist taking into account a number of other factors. The implications of a low AMH level may vary depending upon a woman's age. In younger women a low AMH may indicate that it may be more difficult to obtain eggs during fertility treatment, but does not necessarily mean that eggs obtained from treatment will be poor quality. In other words, while a low AMH indicates a reduced ovarian reserve, it does not necessarily provide information about eggs quality.

What is Dehydroepiandrosterone?

The other treatment related to egg quality that offers help for women dealing with infertility, is DHEA replacement therapy. DHEA is a steroidal hormone that is able to turn into other steroidal hormones (estrogen and testosterone). DHEA is produced mainly from the adrenal glands of young men and women and starts to drop after the age of 30. DHEA has been associated with mental acuity, physical strength, sex drive and memory.[100]

Based upon research conducted by the Center for Human Reproduction in New York, DHEA replacement therapy has been associated with increased embryo counts, embryo quality, and improved fertility treatment as a result. It has decreased miscarriage rates in some women whose primary fertility challenge is Diminished Ovarian Reserve (DOR).

Women, who experience DOR as a result of a slow or inactive adrenal gland and therefore, lack the naturally occurring DHEA, need to be closely monitored when undergoing DHEA replacement therapy. In some instances the treatment rejuvenates ovarian function and increase the chances of pregnancy. Even so, dosage amounts have to be watched closely by your RE because DHEA turns into testosterone and a high level of testosterone can stop ovulation. The effect of DHEA on women with premature ovarian failure, however, still needs more research.[101]

What is DNA Fragmentation Index?

If you and your partner are having trouble conceiving and his semen analysis has come back normal, you may want to talk to your RE about doing a screening for sperm DNA fragmentation. This may render a clearer understanding into why you are not pregnant. A high level of DNA fragmentation may compromise the possibility of natural conception or IUI fertilization outcomes.

The primary function of the sperm is to deliver male DNA to the egg. Therefore the quality of the DNA delivered is tantamount to the development of a healthy embryo. One way to measure the quality and integrity of the DNA is by measuring the fragmented sperm.

If you have ever seen a picture of a sperm it would have been taken through a microscope – they are that small. There is not much to a sperm: a head, a neck and a tail. The head is oval-shaped and this accounts for the main part of the body. The top of the head of the sperm is called an *acrosome*, which contains enzymes that help the sperm penetrate the egg when they meet. The base of the head is called the *post-acrosome*, which is where all the DNA is stored. (Remember the 23 chromosomes?) The neck contains *mitochondria*, which undulates the tail movement so the sperm can swim.

Some sperm are missing the acrosome, so wouldn't be able to penetrate an egg. Some sperm are missing the mitochondria so can't move, though that sperm is still viable. (In other words, though it is not moving it can still fertilize an egg.)

Men produce millions of sperm at a time and they are all in different stages of growth. For an organism that is so small, a sperm performs quite the miracle.

So with research going forward and looking into failed IUI and IVF cycles, a test has been discovered that can look at the DNA of the sperm. This is called the DNA fragmentation test or also called DNA Fragmentation Index (DFI). This test is not part of the general semen analysis. It is a separate test that must be undertaken on its own. The DFI measures the integrity of the DNA in the sperm nucleus, and is associated with a positive or negative pregnancy outcome.

DNA is the hereditary material in humans and other organisms that gives individuals their own characteristics, such as eye color. DNA consists of two long chains or strands that look like a twisting ladder. Genes are the respective parts that compose the ladder. Sometimes, however, part of the ladder breaks or becomes fragmented. This new test DFI can measure the number of DNA fragmented sperm. One of the methods is called the Sperm Chromatin Structure Assay (SCSA), which looks at the sperm's DNA. Approximately 5,000 individual sperm are passed through a high precision flow cytometer, which then measures the sperm for any breaks in the strands of DNA. This renders a DFI score that indicates the likelihood of sperm contributing to infertility problems.

The following scores indicate fertility potential for natural conception and intrauterine insemination:

- Less than or equal to 15 percent DFI: Excellent to Good fertility potential
- 15 percent to 25 percent DFI: Good to Fair fertility potential
- Greater than 25 percent DFI: fair to poor fertility potential

Some doctors suggest that the increase in the DNA-fragmented sperm is the result of reproductive toxins in the environment such as pesticides, insecticides and high levels of air pollution. Other causes can be heat exposure, varicocele, infection, age, smoking, diabetes, testicular cancer, radiation, poor diet and oxidative stress.[102] Obesity also affects the sperm because of the extra stomach weight that insulates the testes, increasing the temperature. Regardless, high DFI affects fertility and increases a recurrence in pregnancy loss.

Having undertaken vigorous research about the causes of increased sperm DFI scores, I wanted to share studies that show how integral the environment and lifestyle choices can elevate the DFI scores. The causes I wanted to examine include: pollution, smoking, oxidative stress, and aging in men.

Teplice, Czech Republic is a town with a heavy winter air pollution generated by burning soft brown coal. Men aged 18, who lived there, underwent a two-year study (spanning the polluted winter and a clean summer), which showed higher than normal infertility and spontaneous miscarriages. The average DFI score was greater than 30 percent, placing them in a group of increased risk for infertility.[103]

It is common knowledge that cigarette smoking is detrimental to health. Recent studies have shown that the components of the cigarette can transfer the blood - testis barrier and contribute to sperm DNA damage through Reactive Oxidative Species (ROS), poor embryo development and development of childhood cancers. In women attempting pregnancy, fertility rate is decreased, early miscarriages are increased and ovarian reserve is altered.[104]

Cigarettes are known source of mutagens and carcinogens and may affect male infertility through elevated sperm DNA fragmentation.

The age of a man has a direct correlation with SCSA defined DFI percentage. In one study, 15 men per decade were enrolled who were characterized by no known infertility issues, were non-smokers, and of similar socio-economic status. Men in their early 20s had an average of approximately five percent DFI, and that value rose about five percent a year. Analysis shows that men at the age of 50 have a one-third chance of having a DFI greater than 30 percent, even if he has fathered children when he was in his twenties. This puts him at a higher risk of infertility and problems fathering a child by natural conception or IUI fertilization. ROS damage is an age related phenomenon and the testis are not an exception.[105]

Recurrent pregnancy loss is a devastating issue for infertility patients. There are many reasons for recurrent pregnancy loss. These include, in part, the age of both partners, though many other reasons mentioned later after IVF. Current research indicates a trend toward increased miscarriages when a high DFI – greater than 30 percent-- is associated with a high rate of miscarriages at 12 weeks of gestation in comparison to the group which had less than 30 percent DFI.[106]

Men, as well as women, are no strangers to the phenomenon of the biological clock ticking away. It's been accepted that the woman's biological clock, when it comes to pregnancy, has been an issue. Now recent studies have shown deterioration of sperm DNA integrity increases with age in men. While it has become socially acceptable to father a child at an older age, this increased age has been shown to correlate with an increased time it takes to be able to get pregnant. Since 1980, U.S. birth rates have increased 40 percent for men 35 to 49 years and have decreased 20 percent for men under 30. Men are having children later on in life as women are too.

What can be done to treat Sperm DNA Fragmentation?

With the development of Intracytoplasmic Sperm Injection (ICSI), some fertility doctors are not as focused on the quality of the sperm generally because a single healthy sperm can be injected into the egg for fertilization.

Where others would like to see the DFI score to come down first and then try natural fertility. If a patient has a varicocele and has it removed, studies have shown not only does it brings the DFI down but can increase pregnancy success. Other ways to decrease the DFI is to eat a healthier diet of fruits and vegetables, eat a diet rich in antioxidants which will help oxidative stress, stop smoking, keep testes cool by avoiding hot tubs, wear boxer shorts and ask your doctor about supplement vitamins and antioxidants like Vitamin E and C and co-enzyme Q-10 and supplements containing carnitine. Men are sperm-banking samples while they in their 30s to use later, in case something happens to their fertility, just as women freeze their eggs at an early age and come back to use those specimens when ready to have family. Maybe this is something to think about!

According to a 2008 report practice committee for the American Society for Reproductive Medicine (ASRM), while there currently is no proven role for routine DNA integrity testing in the evaluation of infertility, sperm DNA damage is more common in infertile men and may affect reproductive outcomes in selected couples, including those with recurrent spontaneous miscarriage or idiopathic (unexplained) infertility. Talk to your RE about having this test performed and it might help explain why you are not having success and maybe there is time to improve the DFI score.[107]

New Test to select the Best Sperm

Researchers are continually discovering ways and techniques to improve the success of IVF. To do this they are attempting to duplicate what really happens in the wonderful miracle of conception inside the body.

Here is a little background on what happens during fertilization: When the egg is ovulated it has a cell membrane around it called the zona pellucida, which is surrounded by a matrix of Hyaluronic Acid (HA). HA is a major component of synovial fluid in your knees and is also good for your skin. Before fertilization, the sperm travel through the fallopian tube, which is undergoing a maturing change to facilitate the sperm's movement. As it travels closer to the egg, the egg attracts the sperm to bind to the zona pellucida. This causes the breakdown and the release of the enzyme in the acrosome (top of the sperm head) to enter the egg (fertilization). This sperm HA interaction completes the natural selective mechanism from the egg to the sperm during fertilization.

According to a study published in the *Journal of Andrology* (June/July, 2010) Dr. Gabor Huszar and his co-workers at Yale University discovered test that isolates sperm with good DNA integrity, a method is comparable to the egg's natural selection.[108]

In the past, a man with a high sperm count and high motility was considered fertile. But this did not include that overall quality of the sperm itself, determining whether or not it could fertilize an egg. In the natural fertilization process the egg selects the optimal mature sperm, but now with IVF and ICSI the whole selection process can be done outside the body. Even so, embryologists have selected sperm to inject into the egg not knowing if it is the optimal sperm.

Huszar has found a biochemical marker, HA, and have tested the idea of binding the sperm to HA. They studied 50 men's samples and the semen was allowed to bind to the hyaluronic acid and these were compared to the original samples. They were able to look at the HA binding sperm and found these sperm possessed very high quality DNA. Those ones that didn't bind possessed DNA fragmentations, which may also carry chromosomal changes that could be related to genetic disorders.[109]

Thus, they were able to identify a key relationship between the ability of sperm to bind to HA and high sperm DNA integrity.

As you can see researchers are looking closely at contingencies related to sperm and finding that this can be contributing to poor fertilization results. Tests like Sperm DNA fragmentation and Sperm binding to HA reflect this ongoing research, highlighting the value of quality sperm optimizing success for normal embryo development. Talk to your RE about these tests and consider looking into them if you are having unsuccessful cycles. The research being done in the area of infertility is quite amazing and the field is constantly changing and improving.

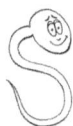

panky says:

"A patient dropped off a semen analysis and said he took some meds accidentally before he collected. I asked him, 'What did you take?' He said, 'Viagra.'"

Chapter 15
The Second Consult

At this point in the process you will meet again with the specialist and review lab and test results and then discuss the plan of action. What happens next? Will you do IUI or IVF?

Keep in mind

As a couple starting in an Infertility program, you are both seeking help. Infertility is a very stressful part of life and as a loving couple who wants to have a family, this is a good time to assess whether or not you are communicating well with one another. It is equally important to resist casting blame on one another if some test results show a problem in one partner. Pointing fingers only increases stress levels. For example, I have heard plenty of times when a couple is dropping off a specimen, perhaps for a second time, and the female will say "It's his fault. He has a low count. I'm fine." I would tell that couple (particularly the female): "Both parties are here for help and the specialist will do his or her best to help. It doesn't help anyone if you start blaming one another."

Let's return to the story about Mary and Tim. When we

last met them, Mary and Tim were in the initial consult in Chapter 8. Now, about two months later, Mary and Tim have had their second consult with the specialist to review the results of their tests. The specialist explains that Mary's Clomid challenge test came out great; her FSH counts were within normal range for this test; and her ovarian reserve and function were fine. High FSH levels are a symptom of DOR (diminished ovarian reserve) or premature menopause. Nevertheless, Mary's hysteroscopy came back with results that reveal a few good-sized uterine fibroids, which could be the reason for her heavy menstrual cycles. Mary's HSG came back normal.[110] The doctor mentions that the fibroids will have to be removed before moving forward and that the nurse will schedule the surgery. Once the fibroids are removed infertility treatment can continue.

As for Tim, his semen analysis results came out fine, though his sperm count was just under normal. The RE did not see any reason why this would impede them from getting pregnant.

Beginning Intrauterine Insemination

The IUI is usually the first plan of action because it is not a surgical procedure, thus less invasive and safer for the patient. It also cost less than IVF. (Many patients may be paying out of pocket for these procedures.)

Before further steps are taken, the RE and/or nurse will review the IUI consent forms with you and you'll sign them. When you enter an infertility program no matter what type of treatment you receive, both parties will have to sign consent forms. The consents will explain the treatment and the potential benefits and risks factors of the treatment. The IUI consent will also cover the medications that you will be on and their risks factors. Most centers try to give the consents ahead of time so you can read them and you will sign them in the presence of your RE and or nurse. This will give you time to ask any questions that you may have before signing.

Despite struggles conceiving they've already experienced, some couples prefer to try a more intentional approach of timed intercourse, on their own, before undergoing any ART (Assisted Reproductive Technique). Depending upon their various test results this could be a workable option. Timed intercourse means the female monitors her ovulation with an ovulation kit. The nurse has instructed the patient when the kit reads positive they should have intercourse that night and the next night. They are to notify their nurse if they don't get a positive reading on the ovulation kit by day 20 or so. If this occurs the nurse will have the patient come in for a blood test to determine whether or not she has ovulated.

Mary and Tim's specialist chooses instead first to undergo an IUI treatment plan for them. He explains the three options (explained in detail below) with needed medications for undergoing an IUI. The doctor hands the couple a sheet that explains the Center's success rate for IUIs over a particular six-month period. The success rate for IUI is 13 to 15 percent. This may sound low, but this is the number of patients pregnant over the total number of cycles, remembering that a single patient may undergo three cycles before success.[111] Many variables contribute to the success rate, such as the age of the patient, uterine factor, PCOS, and male factors. The success rate is also broken down by what medications the patients were taking during that cycle. The success rate will increase when the patient is taking FSH medications. [112]

There are three options to discuss with your RE to begin the IUI treatment. These include: to have no medications, Clomid and FSH injections.

1) No medications

A patient may choose this option if she has never taken fertility drugs and is having trouble figuring out when she is ovulating. The RE will instruct the patient to start testing, using an ovulation test kit on day nine or ten of her cycle. For most women ovulation occurs on days 14 and 15 of the cycle. When the kit registers positive, the patient calls her nurse who will then give instructions for the male partner to drop off a semen sample at the lab the next morning. This sample will then be washed (as described in chapter 17). The female will then come to the center around noon for the IUI procedure.

The hormone being measured in the urine is LH (luteinizing hormone) and this hormone spikes when you are ovulating. Some patients have trouble reading the ovulation kit's results because the result can be a very light colored band on the strip where you put the urine. If this is the case, the hormone can also be measured in the blood and the nurses could have the patient come in daily for LH levels. If you have excellent veins this would not be a problem. But I have seen patients with poor veins, which makes the latter option more problematic.[113]

2) Oral Medication: Clomid

Clomid (Clomiphene citrate) is a medication that stimulates ovulation in women who have infrequent periods or long cycles. Similar to the Clomid challenge test,[114] the patient fills the prescription for Clomid and takes the medication between days five and nine. She will also start with the ovulation kit on days nine or ten. When the ovulation kit turns positive, she will call the nurse and may come in for an ultrasound to see how many follicles are present. In the case of Mary and Tim, the nurse will instruct Mary to have Tim drop off a specimen at the lab the following morning where the semen will be washed. Mary will follow, coming in around noon, for the IUI procedure, receiving the washed specimen. (There is more detail in the IUI section, chapter 17.)

Possible side effects with Clomid are usually mild for most people. As with any medication, however, you should be aware of these before treatment. They include: hot flashes, abdominal pain, headaches, weight gain, mood swings, nausea, dizziness and possibility of twins or multiple births.

3) Injections of FSH (Follicle Stimulating Hormone):

FSH stimulates the ovaries to produce follicles. To maximize the success of IUI or IVF, you want a good number of high quality eggs produced in a month and to have this happen the ovaries need to be stimulated by hormones. Without stimulating medications the ovaries produce only one egg a month. This is where the use of the common medication FSH comes into the picture.

The RE chooses to put the patient on the FSH medications, but it is the nurse who determines which one to order, based upon insurance preference and cost. In states that do not have coverage, the RE may choose one FSH medication over the other out of personal preference. The nurses then will set up the patient both for an injection class to learn self-injection, or, if the center doesn't offer this, they will send the patient home with an instructional DVD that demonstrate how and where to give herself the injections.[115] The injections can be given once or twice daily depending upon the medication she is taking and her particular circumstance. The injection site can be in the stomach or thighs; most women switch off from day to day. The nurses will inform the patient how much of the medication to take and when to take it. Most patients have their partners give the injections. If you have a neighbor or friend who is a nurse, he or she can give the injections. (Next chapter will go into more detail about injections.)

There are side effects to these medications, which can include weight gain, bloating, abdominal discomfort, hot flashes, headaches, ovarian hyperstimulation and "PMS x 1000" (Premenstrual Syndrome: The FSH medications increase the intensity of a normal PMS by a thousand times.)

(I had one patient on the FSH medications who would leave signs in her kitchen to let her husband know to look out! *You know who is back! The B---- is back!*) Patients should always ask their physician about any side effects with medications.

Your nurse will recommend an infertility pharmacy for your medications and many now allow for on-line ordering, which makes it easier for everyone. (Be sure to check with your insurance as they may have selected pharmacies to order from.) These pharmacies are very knowledgeable in the types of drugs you'll be taking and are extremely helpful with questions you may have. The medications can be sent to your home or office and shipping is usually free. (If your insurance covers the medications, the pharmacies will take care of the charges.) You will receive enough medication and related supplies for one month's cycle. Always be aware of your supply in case it becomes low. You don't want unnecessary complications with the process and your cycle.

Monitoring Patients on the FSH medication

Patients who are undergoing an FSH/IUI cycle will generally start on day three of their cycle. When you're on FSH medications the RE will monitor your progress by having blood drawn and transvaginal ultrasounds. FSH medications are a form of estrogen, which stimulates your ovaries to produce follicles. Over time and with more medication, these follicles grow in size and number. The blood is measuring E2 (estradiol), which is a form of estrogen in the body. The FSH medications being injected increase the estrogen levels to help stimulate the ovaries to produce eggs. When the patient has her blood drawn, the test is measuring estradiol and the levels of E2 reflect follicular maturation. These are used along with ultrasound to access the size, number and maturity level of the follicles. This information helps the RE decide the optimal time to perform the IUI procedure.

The blood test is a simple venipuncture and is not difficult for patients who have good veins. There are many patients whose veins are not as easy to find and if the patient's blood is being drawn on a daily basis or every other day for a week or so, this can be unpleasant. One way to avert discomfort is to drink plenty of water all the time, not simply before the blood draw. Your veins will expand with more water intake. In addition, if it is wintertime, be sure your body is plenty warm. On a cold day those veins just disappear.

The blood test is very important so that the RE can monitor you when you start a cycle. No matter what, the technician will need to get that blood. It's a big help for you as the patient to drink water and move around a lot to get those veins popping out.

The transvaginal ultrasound is an imagining technique used to visualize the female reproductive tract. You may remember the ultrasound during which the tech smears gel on your stomach and then uses a hand-held reader. This is still performed in certain ultrasounds, but the transvaginal ultrasounds are more advanced. The transvaginal has a probe that has a condom on it and the technician will give it to you to place in your vagina (you are covered with a sheet). Then the ultrasound technician will guide it to look at the ovaries, count and measure the follicles. One of the ovaries will be dominant because it produces more follicles than the other. This is normal. The ultrasound may be a bit uncomfortable but should not hurt. The ultrasound tech measures the size and number of follicles. As time goes on with more medication, the follicles that increase in size will most likely contain an egg. The ultrasound is also used to measure the thickness of the endometrium (lining of the uterus) and assess its quality for when it is time for implantation.

The nurse schedules each patient in a time slot between 7:00 a.m. and 9:00 a.m. every 15 minutes, so the lab results and ultrasound results can be completed before noontime.

After the doctor has looked at the results and made a determination the nurse will call you that same day with clear instructions. She will tell you to increase your medication or to continue with the same amount. Then she will tell you to come in the next day or that you can skip a day. In any case, she'll book you for another blood draw and ultrasound test and tell you the time to show up for your testing. There might be days when you only have blood work done and no ultrasound, or vice or versa. It's important that you come in the morning and not to miss or be late for an appointment once you begin a cycle with FSH medications. Each visit gives the physician results needed to advance you closer to the ART procedure. (If a day is missed when it's close to your time, a cycle could go too far and be cancelled. Situations do come up and you'll need to call the nurse and hopefully certain arrangements can be made.)

When you are taking the FSH medications, because of the rigorous schedule of blood and ultrasound monitoring, it may be difficult to balance this with the demands of your life. Some couples are very private about infertility and want it kept that way, thus do not want to be explaining lateness to coworkers. Most centers open early, at least by 7:00 a.m., so patients can undergo their tests before they go to work. Our center was a branch of a larger facility based downtown, and patients were very pleased to come here for their testing rather than going into the city, which would have involved a long commute. This may be something to think about when choosing a center: does it have a satellite site close to your work or home? Anything you can do to help reduce the stress is always beneficial.[116]

Some patients will respond well on the injectable FSH medications and produce a number of follicles. A good IUI cycle would consist of at least two to three good-sized follicles. Other patients may respond poorly to the medications and produce very few follicles. Some of the known risk factors for poor response include, older age of the female, obesity, smoking and a history of ovarian surgery. A poor Clomid challenge test can indicate a poor ovarian response to FSH stimulation. Your RE is aware of this and may change medications the following cycle.

When the last day comes and you have two to three follicles that are good size and your E2 result is good, the RE will tell the nurse that you are ready for the IUI procedure. The nurse will call you with instructions to take one more injection. This injection (I used to hear from patients that this is the "Big One") is an intramuscular shot of human Chorionic Gonadotropin (hCG). This shot is given in the buttocks and can hurt. The shot of hCG is given to trigger ovulation, which will occur 30 to 36 hours afterwards. The follicles will open and release the egg. The male partner will go to the lab the next morning and collect a specimen, which will be washed. The female will show up around 11:30 a.m. for the procedure. The sperm will be placed in the uterus and they will swim up to the fallopian tubes waiting to fertilize the released egg.

What is the plan for Mary and Tim?

This being the first time that Mary and Tim have gone to a fertility specialist. Their RE discussed doing three cycles of IUI and taking the oral medication Clomid.

Now that Tim and Mary are in an infertility program, the specialist wants them to have intercourse as much as they want to. However, there are times when the male partner needs to abstain before an IUI procedure so that the sperm sample he produces possesses a good volume and sperm count.

When the RE says three cycles, this means a cycle a month, thus three consecutive months of IUI. If you are still not pregnant, you will make an appointment with your RE for another consult to discuss the next steps. Each RE has his or her own protocol for scheduling consults to keep the plan moving. You are in constant communication with your nurse and she'll guide you.

Chapter 16
Preparing & Giving Yourself Injections

Speaking with couples and asking them what they felt was the most difficult part of the program, they answered surprisingly, the injections! One patient felt that too much time had transpired between the time when they participated in the class to the point at which she needed to start the injection cycle. Another felt the preparation, meaning loading the medication into the syringe, was difficult. Many patients have never given themselves an injection, unless they are diabetic. The process for some can be overwhelming.

Injections for Infertility[117]

It's a painful fact of life that IVF treatment involves giving the woman lots of infertility medications through injection. While most people are naturally needle-phobic, learning how to take these injections yourself can help simplify your life considerably!

If you find the idea of giving yourself a shot more than you can stomach, then you can get your partner to give them to you. (Trust me, no one will give them with more love and care if he messes up, he will never hear the end of it!) And in the process he can learn a new skill as well.

There are basically two types of injections: Intramuscular (IM); and Subcutaneous (SC). Lupron (Buserelin) is usually given subcutaneously; while Menogon (HMG) is usually given intramuscularly. Please remember that there is very little risk of you harming yourself by giving yourself these injections.

It is a good idea to practice on an orange to increase your confidence. You could also ask your nurse to supervise you the first time you give yourself a shot so she can confirm you are doing a good job!

The steps are simple.
1. Assemble your equipment
2. Load the medication into the syringe
3. Prepare the injection site
4. Give the medication
5. Clean up

Find a clean, quiet and comfortable place where you will not be disturbed. Many women find their bathroom or kitchen to be a good spot. Clean a place on the countertop so that you can lay out your supplies. Wash your hands well and dry them thoroughly.

Gather your supplies, including your medications, syringes, needles for mixing drugs (usually bigger) and needles for injecting the drugs (usually smaller), alcohol swabs and sharps container. If you are injecting more than one drug (for example both Buserelin and Menogon) you will want to separate the equipment for one drug from the equipment of the other.

Intramuscular Injections

This type of injection you give into a muscle, which would be given in the buttocks of thigh.

Mixing the diluent and medication

You first need to load the medication into the syringe. You can use a 1 ml or 2 ml syringe. This is usually a simple matter of dissolving the powder with the supplied diluent. Wash your hands and dry them thoroughly.

If your medication comes in rubber-stoppered bottles, you first need to draw up the solvent into a syringe. Remove caps from the rubber stopper vials, which is the dilute vial, and the dry powder medication vial. Wipe the top of the rubber vials with an alcohol swab. Take the cap off the mixing needle (20 gauge) carefully and stick it into the rubber top of vial. Check the diluent and make sure it is clear and nothing is floating in it or it is cloudy (don't use, if so). Make sure you keep the head of the needle under the diluent, do this by bringing the needle down as you aspirate the diluent.

Once you have about 1 ml or 1 cc of diluent using the same needle place the needle in the rubber stopper of the dry powder medicine and add the diluent to the bottle mixing it carefully, do not shake it and be sure to mix it completely, the medication dissolves quickly. Your nurse will instruct you if you need more medication, if so you will add this first mixture to the other dry powder bottles and NOT use any more diluent. (This is very important to get the correct dose of medication)

Usually, one 1 ml of solvent can dissolve up to six vials of the powder. Keeping the diluent volume low will help to reduce the pain of the injection. Use the same procedure as above adding the added medication. Be careful not to stick yourself with the needle, remember it is a sterile needle.

If the medication comes in glass ampules you will need to open the vials by breaking off the glass tops and following the above procedure. Open all the vials at one time to make it easier for yourself.

Once the medication has been loaded into the syringe, remove the 20 G (gauge) needle place needle into sharps container and replace it with a fine 23 G needle. Hold the needle upright and tap the sides of the syringe to make sure there are no air bubbles. Push the plunger every so slight, as to have one drop come out of the syringe again making sure there are no air bubbles present. You can rest the sterile needle back into its cover while you prepare the injection site. Lay the cover on the counter and slide the syringe and needle in the cover.

The injection site

Lying down or standing with your weight off to the side to be injected, locate the upper outer quadrant (or quarter) of your buttock. The injection is given here. The other option is to give it in the outer area of mid-thigh aspect of your thigh, along the middle third. Take a deep pinch between your thumb and forefinger and wipe with alcohol. Then let dry. You should be holding the needle with your dominant hand, once the needle is in use other hand to hold syringe steady and the dominant to push the medicine in.

Place the needle into this pinch of tissue and muscle completely, leaving none of the needle exposed. This ensures you are taking the injection deep into the muscle. Draw back on the plunger. If you are accidentally in a blood vessel (this is highly unlikely) blood will appear in the syringe. If so, pull out the needle, replace it with a new, sterile needle, and repeat the process.

Slowly push the plunger all the way in to inject the medication and then pull the needle straight out. The key to a comfortable injection is swift needle entry followed by slow injection of fluid. Therefore, slowly push the plunger down then quickly withdraw the needle. Alternate between your left and right sides, each time you give yourself an injection. This will prevent the muscles from becoming sore.

Apply pressure and massage the injection site gently for 30 seconds after you administer the shot. Using ice cubes can help to relieve some of the discomfort. Some patients find numbing the skin with ice cubes prior to taking the injection is also helpful before applying alcohol. Never reuse needles and syringes.

Dispose of the syringe in a biohazard container such as a sharps container, which you get from the pharmacy. (Once the container is full, they usually have a mail back program for your container.) Another option is to use an unbreakable plastic container such as a laundry detergent bottle that you can seal and fill half the laundry container with a 1/2 to 1/2 mix of bleach and water. You need to contact your local authority for disposing of the container.

Subcutaneous Injections

A subcutaneous injection is one that is given just under the skin.

Mixing the diluent and medication

You first need to load the medication into the syringe. You usually use a disposable 1 ml insulin syringe. This is usually a simple matter of dissolving the powder in the supplied diluent. Wash your hands and dry them thoroughly.

If your medication comes in rubber-stoppered bottles, you first need to draw up the solvent into a syringe. Remove cap from the rubber stopper from each the dilute vial and the dry powder medication vial. Wipe each rubber cap with alcohol swab. Take the cap of the mixing needle (20 gauge) carefully and stick it into the rubber top of vial. Check the diluent and make sure it is clear and nothing is floating in it (don't use, if so). Make sure you keep the head of the needle under the diluent, do this by bringing the needle down as you aspirate the diluent.

Once you have about 1 ml or 1 cc of diluent using the same needle place the needle in the rubber stopper of the dry powder medicine and add the diluent to the bottle mixing it carefully, do not shake it and be sure to mix it completely, the medication dissolves quickly. Your nurse will instruct you if you need more medication, if so you will add this first mixture to the other dry powder bottles and NOT use any more diluent. (This is very important to get the correct dose of medication.)

Once the medication has been loaded into the syringe, remove the 20 G needle and replace it with a fine 25 G needle. The primary site for a subcutaneous injection is in your abdomen two inches on either side of your navel. Wash your hands thoroughly and make sure that the surface you work on is clean. Sterilize the injection area with an alcohol swab by cleaning about two inches of skin around the injection site. Let it dry for at least one minute. Remove the needle cover. You'll want to hold needle upright and tap the sides of the syringe making sure there are no air bubbles present and again push the plunger ever so slight to have a drop come out of needle ensuring no air is present in syringe.

Pinch the area of skin you have cleansed with alcohol. The injection is given here.

Holding the needle like a pencil about one inch above the injection site, quickly insert the needle. Release the fold of skin. Depress the plunger all the way, injecting all of the medication, and pull the needle straight out. Gently massage the area in circular motion to spread the medication.

Never reuse needles or syringes.

Dispose of the syringes and needles in a biohazard container such as a sharps container or in an unbreakable plastic container such as a laundry detergent bottle that you can see through. Don't try to recap needles, as there is a good chance of sticking yourself. Go to the web sites in the footnotes below and you will see videos, which will help you further along with giving yourself injections.[118]

Helpful tips

1. Your fertility clinic may hold classes on how to do injections. If not, they will be more than happy to show you how to do the first injection. Be sure to ask!

2. If you simply can't bring yourself to give your own injection, see if your partner will do it. If that is not an option, some fertility clinics will do the injections for you for a small fee. (If you're doing daily injections, unless you live nearby your clinic, this might not be practical or check and you may have a nurse in your neighborhood that is willing to help out.)

3. It is normal for some bruising and redness to appear by injection sites, especially if you nick a blood vessel. Try to avoid that area next time you give yourself an injection to avoid further irritation.

4. The possibility exists of contracting an infection at the injection site. Symptoms of an injection infection could be redness and tenderness at the site and a possible fever. You may be instructed to put warm compresses (face clothes) at the site and be put on antibiotics.

5. Some patients will put ice on the area for the injection for a few minutes prior to injection. This will

help numb the site.

6. Breathe, don't rush and remember: the first time is the most difficult! You don't know what to expect and it may feel crazy to be aiming a needle at your tummy. Trust me – after the first time it gets much easier.

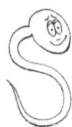 panky says:

"A patient called to book a Semen Analysis and I said that he should be two to four days abstinent for the specimen. He said, 'I know. I'm on day three, so I hope I don't see a pretty girl before that!'"

Chapter 17
What is the procedure for an IUI?

Many patients are self-conscious about dropping off their semen specimen at the lab for washing. Will many other patients be there? (Some fear embarrassment and others are worried if someone else is there that may know them.) How can I feel assured that we are getting my (washed) specimen back?

The lab I managed had very strict training procedures, which were carefully thought through at every step to ensure that there were no problems or mix-ups. Our standard procedure dictates that we worked with only one specimen out at a time and that all the equipment for the procedure was sterile and disposable so as not to taint or distort the results. I would speak freely with patients about their discomfort and as time went on they began to feel a trusting relationship with the staff and became very comfortable. Any professional working in this field will assure all their patients that their top priority is to be certain that the couple will get back their own washed specimen. It is my hope that after reading this book, patients will clearly understand what happens in an infertility program and thus will feel more at ease.

Always feel free to ask any questions; there are no ridiculous questions.

Depending upon what medication protocol the doctor has assigned, the nurses will instruct the patient on the step-by-step implementation of the upcoming procedure. If she is not on a medication or taking Clomid and instead using an ovulation kit, the nurse will still be involved. The patient will call the nurses if the test registers positive to let them know the result.[119]

If you are doing FSH injections you have come in for about a week and a half of ultrasounds and blood work. This could be a total of five to seven visits during that time; depending upon how quickly your E2 increases and the follicles increase in size. You have spoken to the nurse when the RE decided that you are ready and you have taken the shot of hCG the night before and your partner is to drop a specimen off the next morning.

The female partner will come back the same day around 11:30 a.m. or 12:00 noon and go to the lab to pick up the specimen and will be shown where to go for the procedure.

It is very important that the male partner brings a government photo ID (driver's license or passport) to show the laboratory. Most labs will ask for this and depending on their policies may not do the procedure if a photo ID is missing. (I continue to be astonished at how many people drive around leaving their licenses at home.) I know some folks may need to dash out of the house because the procedure is scheduled for the morning and are rushing to get the specimen to the lab. But don't forget a photo ID. In most cases the lab only allows a drop off by the male partner so a proper identification can be made and the specimen cup has to be labeled with full name and date of birth of the male partner.

We did have an occasion where the male partner was so nervous about dropping off; he gave the bag with the specimen in it to another employee and left the building. The specimen was not labeled but there was some paperwork in the bag, which told us the specimen, was intended for a semen analysis. Because of the inability to confirm the specimen source, the patient was called to come back and recollect. The original specimen would be disposed of.

When the male partner submits a specimen he will fill out a drop-off sheet, which includes his and his partner's names and dates of birth. (Make sure you know it!) He signs the intake form, which confirms that the specimen he is giving is his. He will also be asked how many days of abstinence since the last time he ejaculated. An IUI sample should have between two to four days abstinence. If he had intercourse the night before giving a sample the next morning, the specimen will show a low volume and low sperm count. The body needs to build it back up. If it has been more than seven days abstinence, that too may result in a high non-motile sperm count, which may be difficult to remove from the wash. It is optimal to strike the right balance. Abstain long enough to build up healthy sperm, while also "cleaning the pipes" to get rid of the non-motile sperm. So it is important to try to keep the days in order (as mentioned, between two and four) so there can be a good sample to wash for the IUI.[120]

The specimen has to be washed before it can be transferred into the female's uterus. Each lab has a different method of performing the washing procedure. The specimen is usually put on different layers of gradient. Gradients have different viscosities so they don't mix, like water and oil. When the semen is put on top of the gradient, it forms like a kind of "net" between itself and the semen. When the specimen is centrifuged the netting will hold back the non-motile sperm and contents of the semen. This centrifugation separates the motile from non-motile sperm, removes prostaglandins and any viscosity to the specimen. (Some women may get some cramping after intercourse, which may be caused by these prostaglandins in the semen.) The wash improves the specimen and the IUI puts the healthier fast-moving sperm closer to its destination. The lab will perform a sperm count before and after the wash, which will be documented on patient's chart. A good sperm wash will result in an improved percentage of motile sperm.

After the specimen has been delivered and washed, the female partner comes in at a certain time (around 11:30) to pick up the now-washed specimen that is in a sterile plastic tube and labeled with her partner's name, date of birth, or medical record number. The tube has about ½ ml of specimen, which at the time of ovulation is the proper amount for the uterus to take in. A good sperm count will cause the specimen to be hazy or cloudy in appearance. The lab technician will sign off the specimen and the female partner needs to show a government photo ID. The technician will tell the patient that the specimen needs to be kept warm until the insemination. To insure this, she might put the tube down her bra or at the top of her pants. The technician will direct her to the office where the IUI procedure is performed.

She will be called in to an exam room (her partner is welcome to join). For some couples the first IUI may feel unusual, less intimate. To help his partner feel more intimate about it, some men bring a long stem rose. The male partner will be with his partner at the head of the exam table during the procedure. The RE will review the identification of the specimen with the patient and he or she will take the specimen and place it in a catheter. An IUI is very similar to getting a pap smear. A speculum is placed inside the vagina and the catheter is placed through the patient's cervix. The specimen will be injected into the uterus. Then the patient relaxes on the exam table for about 10 minutes. Check with the nurse, but usually after this brief recovery time the patient is set to return to her normal routine.

The cervix is the lower, narrow portion of the uterus where it joins with the top end of the vagina. The cervix has an opening, which in most women is usually located in its center. When the specialist examines inside the vaginal canal he or she is looking for the cervix opening, which is in the center of the cervix (resembles a doughnut) and this allows passage to the uterus. This opens only during ovulation and the menstrual cycle. In some women the cervix opening is not centered and is in the upper left or right corner, when this happens the specialist may need to work on getting the catheter through the opening, so it can be uncomfortable for a brief period of time.

The cervix can be vascular so some women may get some spotting and cramping after the procedure. This is considered normal.

Some centers do two IUIs, one on one day and the other the next day. Other centers will perform only one. Sperm can live up to five days in the female, depending on the environmental conditions. Timing is everything getting the little swimmers up there to meet the egg(s).

The patient can ask for the sperm count before and after the wash so that she can tell her partner. The majority of sperm samples are improved after the wash. By doing an IUI, the lab is making the specimen better (depending on what they are given).[121] Beyond that, the sample has less area to travel to reach the egg by placing it directly into the uterus, though it still has to travel up the fallopian tubes to the released egg(s).

Patients are put on progesterone supplements the day after the IUI to help thicken the uterine lining for implantation. The progesterone comes in a vaginal suppository or can be taken by IM (Intramuscular) injection.

The nurses will tell the patient to call the center and come in for a pregnancy test if she does not get her menstrual cycle within two weeks (14 days) from the IUI procedure.

If the patient gets her menstrual cycle and is on FSH medications, she will need to call the nurse, who will set an appointment for a baseline ultrasound and have blood drawn for hormones. The baseline ultrasound is looking for any cysts on the ovaries and it should register negative (meaning no cysts) before you move on to the next cycle. This ultrasound usually takes place during the menstrual cycle.[122] The FSH medication may cause cysts on the ovaries and if the cysts are present it will be necessary to skip a month before starting the next cycle to allow this type of cyst to disappear on its own. The patient will have a follow-up ultrasound to double check before starting the next cycle.

Possible Complications and Risks after a FSH / IUI

1. Different Responses to FSH Medications

Women's ovaries may respond differently to the FSH stimulation medications. Some women may not respond at all and thus not produce any follicles. Whereas others respond too much and get over stimulated and produce too many follicles for an IUI procedure. Lest you be confused, we want many follicles when the patient is to undergo an IVF cycle because the eggs are removed from your body. But in the case of an IUI, the eggs remain in the body, so each follicle has the potential to become a fetus.

This is when the RE makes a decision and speaks to the patient to see about an IVF conversion. This means the patient can transition from the simpler IUI phase to the major stage of the IVF. The nurse will speak to the patient's insurance company about converting this cycle to an IVF (In Vitro Fertilization) cycle. If a patient is allowed to covert to an IVF, it is exciting to reach this stage since she has reached the final stage without having to do anything extra. Her body produced too many eggs.

If the patient is not allowed to move on to IVF or is paying out-of-pocket this would mean the cycle might be cancelled because of the cost. The RE stops the cycle because he/she does not want his patient to have multiple births, which could mean greater than three to four babies. Anytime the patient goes through infertility there is chance of multiple births, but the RE is trying to keep control of the number of births. When the cycle is stopped it is not without reason. Your RE will gain more knowledge of your infertility and will make changes for future cycles. So don't get discouraged. Every patient can react differently on these FSH medications.

2. Body Ovulates on its own before IUI procedure:

Another situation that can occur while taking the FSH medications is that some women could ovulate on their own before the follicles are ready. Your RE is timing everything, but there is a chance that the body could ovulate, opening the follicles and releasing the egg and the E2 drops before the IUI procedure has commenced. The RE would tell the patient to have intercourse that evening, with the hope of getting pregnant. If this occurs the cycle is cancelled because there will be no eggs to fertilize. The opportunity is missed. To help prevent this from happening in the next cycle, the RE may put the patient on Lupron, a medication that is used for IVF cycles that prevents premature ovulation. It would be an added injection to your FSH regimen but it should help in the future cycle.

3. Ovarian Hyperstimulation (OHSS)

There is a complication that women can develop when taking the FSH medications and it is called OHSS (Ovarian hyperstimulation syndrome). It can develop after taking the FSH medication that acts directly on your ovaries stimulating them to produce multiple eggs.

OHSS is a severe complication that can arise from taking the FSH medications. It usually occurs after the injection of the trigger shot hCG. Signs and symptoms usually appear 10 days after the trigger injection of hCG when the ovarian blood vessels have an abnormal reaction to the hormone and begin to leak fluid. This fluid can swell the ovaries and sometimes moves into the abdomen in large amounts. The syndrome is characterized by ovarian enlargement and abdominal/gastrointestinal discomfort. The severity is graded on the basis of the size of the ovaries, subjective complaints, and laboratory/radiologic findings.

There are mild, moderate, and severe cases of OHSS. Most women have a mild-to-moderate case. (If a women has OHSS she will have symptoms, but for some women these may not be as severe.) The patient will have blood work, ultrasounds and be told to drink plenty of fluids like Gatorade. Patients may complain of pain, a bloated feeling and mild abdominal swelling, which will invariably resolve within a few days unless pregnancy occurs. If you are pregnant your body is producing the hormone hCG and the symptoms can last longer in the beginning of your pregnancy. OHSS will be explained in more detail in the IVF risk section of the book.

4. Multiple Pregnancies

The RE does his/her best to monitor the patient's cycle and determines whether or not, and when to trigger the cycle. It is possible to have multiple follicles present that can get fertilized and subsequently implant in the uterus. If there are multiple follicles that are large enough and can have an egg, there is no control on how many will fertilize and thus, how many will be implanted. The number of fetuses will be discovered at the ultrasound, which will occur about five weeks after the IUI procedure.

5. Ectopic Pregnancy (Tubal Pregnancy)

The ultrasound that is given at five weeks to determine the number of fetuses is also looking to rule out an ectopic pregnancy. The fetuses are implanted in the uterus. But sometimes they implant in the fallopian tubes. There is a five percent possibility that an ART procedure can end up in an ectopic pregnancy, which some may resolve itself through spontaneous abortion or will be corrected with medication or surgery. (Ectopic pregnancy will be further discussed in IVF section.)

To review: One cycle is a month long and, depending on your RE's plan, the patient would undertake three consecutive months of the IUI treatment. If pregnancy has not resulted after that time, the patient will meet with the RE for another consult. Together they will review the previous cycles and look at the sperm results after the sperm wash and consider the next step. This is a good time for the patient to speak honestly with the RE and bring up anything at all that may be confusing or upsetting. Depending upon what medication she was on for the first set of three cycles, the medical team may change to an alternative medication. For example if the patient took Clomid for the first set, and it wasn't effective, then she may be moved to the FSH injectables for the next set. If she has insurance that covers infertility generally, they may suggest undergoing a certain number of IUIs before moving to the IVF procedure. If she can get pregnant doing IUI, it is less expensive than IVF and thus worth the extra effort.

If you have to pay out of pocket expense for the IUI procedure, prices can vary between one infertility clinic to the next. For example, the FSH medication could cost up to $1,000 - $2,000 per month and the procedure for IUI is over $1,500.

panky has a story:

"A female patient got stopped for speeding on her way to our lab. She showed the officer the specimen cup and told him where she was going and he let her go right along. I found out later that the policeman was also a patient and completely understood. But don't drive too fast. The specimen is fine as long as it is kept at body temperature and delivered within 45 minutes from the time of collection."

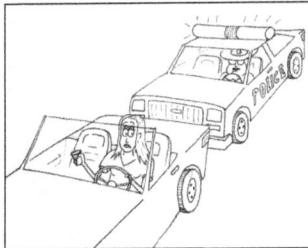

Chapter 18
In Vitro Fertilization (IVF)

In Vitro Fertilization is a process wherein the egg cells are fertilized by sperm outside the body. IVF is a major last-resort treatment for infertility after all other methods of ART (Assisted Reproductive Technologies) have failed. During the IVF cycle, the process overrules other natural contingencies (such as natural ovulation) in deference to the larger goal of achieving controlled fertilization and hopefully pregnancy.

The process involves hormonally controlling the female's ovaries to produce eggs, which are manually removed from the ovaries to be fertilized by washed sperm in a fluid medium outside the body. The fertilized egg (embryo) is then transferred back into the patient's uterus with the hope of producing a sustainable pregnancy. The first successful procedure of this nature was the birth of a "test tube baby," Louise Brown, born in 1978. Most patients resort to an IVF cycle after they have had a number of failed IUI attempts using Clomid and FSH medications. IVF is more expensive than an IUI because it involves an actual surgical procedure.

During the earliest years of IVF treatment, couples en-

tered the process understanding that this was a procedure that, because of scientific advancement, produced
an embryo outside of the body (in a petri dish). This inevitably, created a dilemma on many levels, morally,
religiously or ethically, or all of the above. At the same
time, these couples desperately wanted children and had
not had success conceiving "the old fashion way." They
needed assistance. As a result of this complicating aspect
of the treatment, two procedures were developed that
allowed for medical intervention while at the same time
keeping the natural process as far as was possible. These
procedures are called Gamete Intrafallopian Transfer
(GIFT) and Zygote Intrafallopian Transfer (ZIFT).

GIFT (Gamete Intrafallopian Transfer): This is very much
like IVF except that when the eggs and sperm are put
together, instead of leaving them in a petri dish for fertilization, are placed in the fallopian tubes using a laparoscopic procedure. (In the IVF procedure the embryos are
incubated three to five days before being transferred directly into the uterus.) The GIFT technique follows nature
by allowing fertilization to occur inside the female's body
and the embryo implants naturally. GIFT is a favorable option, depending on one's ethical concerns about infertility
treatment because it enables the patient to undergo an
ART procedure without the moral dilemma concerning
the number of embryos to transfer back in to the female.

ZIFT (Zygote Intrafallopian Transfer): The female's eggs
are mixed with the sperm of the male partner in a dish in

the embryology lab. The fertilized eggs, called zygotes, are then transferred within 24 hours into the fallopian tubes. (In the IVF procedure the embryos are incubated three to five days before being transferred directly into the uterus.) ZIFT can be more successful than GIFT because the embryologist knows they are transferring already-fertilized eggs.

The main difference between GIFT and ZIFT lies in the fact that the former GIFT transfers a random mixture of sperm and eggs (before fertilization) to the fallopian tubes; whereas the latter, ZIFT, transfers a fertilized egg(s) directly into the fallopian tubes. These procedures are generally used when a couple's religious or ethical constraints forbid in vitro fertilization. In general the success rate of general IVF (without GIFT or ZIFT) tends to overrule those who opt for these other procedures, making them less common. In any case, a women is able to consider these procedures only if she possesses healthy fallopian tubes.

Let's return to the case of Mary and Tim. They went through three IUI cycles using Clomid and three cycles with FSH over a period of nine months, none of which resulted in a pregnancy. (Remember, Mary developed cysts on her ovaries, which meant they had to skip a month or two.)[123] After having had a consult with their RE, together they made the decision to move on to IVF for the next phase of infertility treatment. The nurses have contacted Mary's insurance company and verified her coverage for IVF. The insurance company says Mary has a "Life Time" maximum of $45,000 for IVF treatment. The price of a typical IVF cycle would allow Mary to undergo three IVF cycles.[124]

IVF Consent Forms

Consent forms will need to be signed before beginning an IVF cycle. Your nurse will give the couple a packet of consent forms to read and sign at some point before the procedure. Consent forms must be signed in the office in the presence of the nurse or RE. There are many ART procedures that can be performed as part of IVF, or performed on their own, some of which may or may not occur at this phase. It is a good idea for the couple to read carefully all the consents and then raise any questions before the procedure at a follow-up meeting with the RE. Here is the breakdown of the procedures and the consents that may be needed to sign:

IVF and other ART Procedures

1. IVF: As noted, this is the most successful ART procedure and is usually performed after patients have had no success with IUI procedures. Some REs will opt to skip the IUI altogether if, for example, the male partner has a very low sperm count or low motility, or there are other complicating issues of infertility.

The consent forms go over risk factors and options that exist for embryos that are not transferred back to the female and may not be of a quality viable enough to freeze.

2. ICSI (Intracytoplasmic Sperm Injection): Some couples may need additional help in fertilizing the eggs, in

which case ICSI is performed. This procedure involves the sperm being injected directly into the egg to cause fertilization. It is performed on patients whose male partner has a very low sperm count or very low motile sperm count. It is also performed on patients with poor fertilization results. In a typical IVF procedure the sperm and eggs are put together in a petri dish where they are left to fertilize on their own. (Sometimes it can happen that not all the eggs fertilize, no eggs fertilize, or the quality of the fertilized egg is poor, then this would be considered poor fertilization results.) After the ICSI procedure the injected egg and sperm are left to incubate in the petri dish and will be viewed in a day or two for fertilization results.

3. Assisted Hatching: For couples who have had a number of failed IVF cycles, the next procedure the RE will suggest is Assisted Hatching. This is a very fragile procedure that involves making small hole in the outer covering of the embryo, called the zona pellucida, which speeds up the process of the zona hatching. The process of Assisted Hatching creates an opening in the zona pellucida making it easy for embryo to escape, or hatch, and attach or implant in the uterus. Assisted Hatching is performed just prior to the embryo transfer. (This is procedure is performed only after more than one failed IVF cycles.)

4. Embryo Cryopreservation (Freezing Embryos): If, after the IVF procedure, there remain many embryos of good quality and graded highly, the embryologists looks at the petri dishes under the microscope after the sperm

and egg have incubated for at least two days, they assign them a grade that relates to the quality of the embryo. Statistically high quality embryos are more successful for a pregnancy. Some patients when they do an IVF cycle produce around 20 eggs. If most of these become fertilized and have good-grading results, then freezing some embryos for a future cycle is a great option. The embryology lab freezes the embryos through a process in which the embryos stay frozen (sometimes for months and even for years)[125] until the couple is ready to try another cycle. During this cycle, which called a frozen cycle, the patient takes fewer medications then a typical IVF cycle because there is no stimulating the ovaries to produce more eggs, only preparing the uterus for an embryo transfer. A number of embryos are thawed in an incubator and transferred into the uterus just like a typical IVF transfer. The couple has the final authority as to the disposition of the cryopreserved embryos.

5. Consents for Medications:[126]Ovarian stimulation or Super ovulation drugs are used to induce the patient's ovaries to grow several mature eggs rather than the single egg that normally develops each month. This regimen is done because the chances for pregnancy are increased if more than one egg is fertilized and transferred to the uterus in a treatment cycle. Depending upon the program and the patient, both the drug type and the dosage varies. Most often the drugs are given over a period of nine to twelve days. Drugs currently in use include: Human Menopausal Gonadotropin (HMG), Follicle Stimulating

Hormone (FSH), Human Chorionic Gonadotropin (HCG) and gonadotropin releasing hormone (GnRH) agonists. The following explains what the medications are used for:

- Human Menopausal Gonadotropin (HMG): Some women are put on this medication because they don't ovulate on their own and have pituitary deficiencies with hormone production. This medication contains FSH and LH and will stimulate ovaries to produce follicles.
- Follicle Stimulating Hormone (FSH): This medication is used to stimulate the ovaries to produce follicles.
- Gonadotropin Releasing Hormone (GnRH) agonists: This medication, called Lupron, is given so women won't ovulate during the IVF cycle. The medication suppresses the pituitary gland so the RE can induce follicle growth with FSH medication.
- Human Chorionic Gonadotropin (HCG): This is the intramuscular shot you take after you have taken HMG or FSH medication, which triggers the follicle to open and release the egg.

Mock Embryo Transfer

At some time before the true IVF cycle Mary will schedule a mock embryo transfer with the RE, which can be done in the office. The purpose is to measure the angle and depth of the patient's cervix, uterus and the thickness of her uterine lining. The mock transfer process helps to ensure the actual embryo transfer proceeds smoothly, optimizing the embryo implantation. The embryo transfer itself is performed with ultrasound but the mock transfer will help with any difficulty that can unexpectedly arise. So this procedure eliminates potential problems that may arise when you undergo your first IVF cycle.

The nurse will set this up and it needs to be performed prior to the cycle. The mock embryo transfer involves inserting a catheter into the uterus and recording the length of the catheter and any special twists or turns that it takes to get the catheter smoothly inserted. There are different catheters that could be used. The trial procedure enables the team to determine which one is best. This procedure is part of the preparation for the real embryo transfer enabling the RE to circumvent potential problems.

Ovarian Stimulation: Taking the Injection Medications

After the RE reviews the test results—including the patient's age, medical history of ovulation, and ovarian reserve—they then begin a hormonal protocol of the appropriate medications to stimulate the ovaries.

There are different types of medications, each with its own purpose and intended goal. For example, during a typical IVF cycle, if the patient isn't ovulating on her own, the RE will put her on a HMG injection along with Lupron. On the other hand, if she is ovulating on her own the RE will put her on a FSH medication and Lupron. In both cases the HCG will be taken at the end of the cycle to trigger ovulation.

The goal of ovarian stimulation for IVF is to be able to retrieve approximately eight to 15 quality eggs to be removed from the ovaries. The medication stimulates the ovaries to produce multiple follicles over a single month. Finding the right balance of stimulation is tricky because each patient responds differently to the ovarian stimulation protocols. Some may respond by producing too many follicles[127] and others may produce only a few follicles or none at all. The RE will be unable to make this determination until the patient starts her cycle. Success can occur in IVF even with a low number of eggs retrieved. Obviously, success rates increase substantially when more eggs are recovered.[128]

If, after having undergone an IVF cycle, and the patient responds poorly to the medications and produces a low number of follicles, the RE may begin what is called a Flare protocol or a short protocol.[129] A Flare protocol could also be assigned to patients who have responded poorly and did not produce a good number of eggs.

The Flare protocol involves Lupron being started earlier in the cycle, which precipitates an initial "flare-up" response of FSH and LH release from the woman's pituitary gland, which the RE wants to harness. This usually occurs in the first three days of the Lupron administration. It is a kind of "jump start" for the ovaries to produce more follicles. You may also be put on birth control pills the month before this type of stimulation.[130]

Beginning the IVF Cycle

To begin the standard IVF cycle, which is a longer protocol than a Flare, the RE needs to determine a starting point in her cycle (detailed below).[131] To locate the starting point of a cycle, going back to Mary and Tim, the nurse will schedule Mary to come in on day 21 of her next cycle. (This should be far enough along after Mary ovulated that month, probably around day 14.) Mary will come in for a blood test to measure progesterone levels since rises in the blood after ovulation. The RE likes to see a result greater than 4 nanograms. If the results determine that Mary has ovulated, the medication protocols can begin. (If the results reflect progesterone levels that are not high enough, the nurse will have Mary return in a couple of days for a second progesterone test.)

Once progesterone levels indicate that Mary has ovulated naturally she will be instructed to start taking injections of Lupron, which will prevent the body from ovulating naturally in the upcoming cycle. This initiates the protocols that will "take over" the body's hormonal functions until completion of the IVF cycle.

Though this sounds odd and even contradictory, IVF has its own logic. The goal of IVF is facilitate the female producing as many eggs as possible. To facilitate this, the RE wants to control egg production by means of FSH and then manually retrieve the ripe and healthy eggs to continue the process of fertilization outside the body. It might help to think of it this way: during an IVF cycle the medications take over the bodily production of eggs. Part of this is taking Lupron to avoid any spontaneous release of the egg naturally, which could potentially derail the controlled procedure. The RE wants to know when the time is right to harvest hormonally produced eggs, and any naturally released eggs would sabotage the process.

It is also important that the patient avoid intercourse at this point, for similar reasons. Because the cycle started around day 21, which is luteal phase (the time just after ovulation and before the menstrual cycle). During this phase of the cycle the potential exists for the already-released egg to become fertilized, which would similarly derail the highly controlled IVF cycle. Couples should avoid unprotected intercourse in this cycle.[132]

Mary will also be instructed to take her injections of FSH. At this point she will be taking up to two shots a day, if not more.

She will come in for blood and ultrasounds as directed by her nurse. The bloods will be measuring the E2 (estradiol) and ultrasounds will measure the number and size of follicles. This part of the protocol involves a few more blood samples and ultrasounds, then the FSH IUI – again because the specialist wants as many follicles as possible to be produced. The nurse will call Mary each day during this process to render instructions according to her results. She may continue with the same amount or possibly increase medications. She will also book the next appointment for more blood work and ongoing ultrasounds.

After approximately 10 to 12 days of the gonadotropin (FSH) injections, the follicles will almost be mature. When the ultrasound scan indicates a reasonable size and number of follicles and the diameter of the leading follicles is greater than 16 mm; and if the E2 (estradiol) levels are increasing along with size of follicles; and, assuming the RE feels that the patient has met the criteria for egg retrieval;

he/she will trigger the cycle with the HCG injection. The nurse will call with specific instructions about what time to take the injection of HCG, which finalizes growth and maturation of the eggs. The nurse will also tell the patient to stop all other injections and give her the date and time for her surgery.

Your partner should have two to three days of abstinence on the day of the surgery. There should be no intercourse during the time after the HCG injection and 48 hours after the procedure.

The ultrasound result indicates that Mary has 13 follicles that are good sized for the retrieval (five on the left ovary and eight on the right). In addition, the lining of the womb (endometrium) shows a good thickness, which is good for implantation of the embryos.

Ovulation takes place 30 to 36 hours after the HCG injection. Timing is critical. Mary might be scheduled possibly in the midst of other patients' procedures at different times and a patient might be instructed to take the HCG medication at 11:00 a.m. or 12:00 p.m.

The surgical procedure for removing the eggs is called Egg Retrieval and this occurs two days after taking the shot of HCG. Mary was told to take her injection at 12 midnight on a Sunday. She will thus be scheduled to have her IVF procedure Tuesday before 12 noon.

It was mentioned earlier that if a patient produces a high number of follicles an IUI cycle could be converted to an IVF cycle. Well, the same is true conversely. An IVF cycle could be converted to an IUI cycle if a patient doesn't produce enough follicles or if the blood E2 (estradiol) level drops. (If this occurs the RE may tell the couple to have intercourse that night and come in the next day for an IUI.) Each patient is different and thus the process doesn't necessarily follow the same book, so to speak. Don't get discouraged. Each cycle gives the specialist added information that will inform changes and adaptation for the next cycle.

What should Mary expect on the retrieval day?

IVF is a surgical procedure for which Mary will be given an anesthesia. She will have to abstain from eating and drinking for eight to ten hours beforehand. Upon arrival at the clinic the nurse in the Embryology department will meet her and answer any questions she may have. The nurse will start an IV (intravenous) line in her arm for administering medication. The anesthetist will review Mary's medical history before starting the sedation medication.

Once Mary is medicated the procedure will begin. Retrieval can take up to 30 to 45 minutes. The most common technique is using a vaginal ultra sound probe which has a fine hollow needle attached to it. Under ultrasound guidance, the needle will enter each follicle and drain the fluid out. An embryologist then evaluates the follicular fluid and finds the eggs. (All of this evaluation is done under a microscope where the eggs have been placed in a petri dish along with culture media.)[133]

After the procedure Mary may notice some cramping similar to menstrual cramping. Tylenol is usually sufficient to relieve any discomfort.[134]

While Mary is in the retrieval, Tim will be called into

the Embryology collection room to collect his specimen. The embryology lab will wash Tim's specimen. A fresh semen specimen is always best for the IVF procedure. Some male partners "sperm-bank" their own specimen in the event something (such as travel) might cause them to be unavailable on the day of the retrieval. Further, it is there as a backup specimen if, on retrieval day, the male experienced performance anxiety or low sperm count. In those cases the IVF lab could be using a frozen semen specimen. (This will be explained more in the Sperm bank section). Some men may be having a testicular biopsy to retrieve the sperm and this would happen at the same time as the egg retrieval. The sperm will be placed with the eggs about three to six hours after the retrieval.

When the retrieval is completed the patient will take one to two hours for recovery. The nurse will give discharge instructions and the RE will start her on a medication regimen, including an antibiotic to prevent infection, a steroid to reduce any inflammation in the reproductive organs, and progesterone hormonal supplements. The progesterone prepares the lining of the uterus for implantation and keeps the lining thick, which is needed for a successful pregnancy. Some facilities start the progesterone the day after the retrieval.

Some patients take progesterone by IM (intramuscular) injection or by taking suppositories. (Patients may prefer one or the other for their own reasons.) In any case, it is important to take this hormone since it increases the success with IVF. She will continue it daily for the next two weeks according to the schedule she will have received.

The progesterone is usually taken nine to ten weeks into the pregnancy, until the placenta takes over and starts producing it on its own.

The patient may be asked to refrain from sexual intercourse for a period of time or to avoid submerging herself in water (such as taking a bath). She will need to use a pad, not tampons, to address any light bleeding that sometimes occurs in the weeks following egg retrieval. (If this is the case it is imperative to call the RE promptly.) Other symptoms include:

- Low abdominal discomfort, pain or bloating
- Shortness of breath
- Weight increase of two to three pounds a day
- Decreased urine output and painful urination
- Running a fever above 101 degrees F.
- Heavy vaginal bleeding (soaking through a pad in an hour, some light bleeding is normal)
- Fainting or dizziness

The symptoms can occur up to two weeks after egg retrieval. It is common to have a sensation of heaviness or cramping in your pelvis for four to ten days after egg retrieval. Your ovaries frequently enlarge at this time.

What happens next to the eggs and sperm?

The embryologists will take care of the eggs, sperm and soon-to-be embryos in the lab. An embryologist is a scientist who studies the formation, early growth and development of living organisms. Clinical embryologists work with human embryos, as opposed to non-clinical embryologists, who work with animal and plant embryos.

For a couple struggling with infertility the embryologist in the IVF lab plays a vital role in the journey to pregnancy. The major responsibilities of the embryologists in the chain of command is to make sure that all specimens belong to the correct patients and that all samples that are put together are from the correct patients. (There are always two embryologists identifying samples of retrieved eggs, semen samples and petri dishes that are labeled with couple's identification.) The other part of their job is to prepare the embryology lab by regulating and testing environmental conditions, including temperature, air quality, and humidity. The embryologist is the person who takes the eggs at the time of retrieval and puts them in petri dishes along with a culture media (which resembles the fluid in a female's uterus) and places specimens in incubators. A few hours later they add the washed sperm to the petri dishes and let the normal fertilization process begin.

Mary's eggs will be placed in a petri dish along with Tim's sperm. There may be more than one petri dish, depending on the number of eggs retrieved. The petri dish(s) are properly labeled with the couple's names and dates of birth and will be placed in a well-monitored incubator on different shelves. During that time the sperm will fertilize the eggs and the eggs will be examined for fertilization results by the embryologist. The nurse will call Mary with her fertilization results on the next day after the retrieval. Fertilization is when the sperm enters the egg and this stage is called a zygote and the embryologist can see this stage under the microscope. They will count and see how many eggs were able to fertilize and this is what they report out as fertilization results. The zygote becomes an embryo as it furthers develop. These embryos are viable and will stay in the petri dish and are graded by the embryologist for quality. The embryos with the good quality will be placed back into the uterus during the IVF transfer or – depending upon the number-- some may be able to be frozen for a future cycle.

Intracytoplasmic Sperm Injection (ICSI)

For some patients, when the male has very low sperm counts, very low motile sperm, or a very high abnormal morphology result, the RE will recommend ICSI. This option is introduced as well for a couple that previously has had low fertilization results or failed previous IVF cycles. We had a patient that had no motile sperm whatsoever and underwent ICSI, which resulted in a beautiful boy. The embryologist looks for the mature eggs and then picks up a sperm with a needle and injects it into the egg. This is done with the help of a tool called a manipulator, which is connected to the microscope. (All of this being done under the microscope.) Once the eggs are retrieved the ICSI procedure starts within a few hours. The procedure is completed when the eggs have been injected with sperm and are placed in the incubator.

Regardless of the method of fertilization (IVF or IVF-ICSI), the petri dishes remain in a controlled environment in the incubator within a culture medium for a couple of days to be observed for fertilization results and grading.

There are many embryo-grading systems that differ in how they assign "grades" to the quality of the embryo. The embryo grading systems are subjective. Some labs grade the embryos on day two or day three. This grading system help the embryologists determine the quality of the embryos according to certain guidelines, which informs their determining what embryos can be transferred and frozen. (A further explanation of the grading system is discussed below.) The quality of the fertilization is important because the better the quality the better chances for a successful pregnancy.

In the early days of IVF, the thinking was that embryos would do better being transferred shortly after fertilization. With the improvement of lab culture media, embryos can remain in culture a day or two longer so that the embryologist can determine which embryos are growing most robustly. A day-3 embryo has eight cells, so any embryos at the same stage that contain fewer cells would not be chosen. Embryos stay in the incubator for at least three days and maybe up to five days before they are transferred to the recipient.

What is the Embryologist looking for?

The embryologist will look at the petri dishes under the microscope and see how many eggs fertilized and grade each one of them according to quality of their appearance, cell number and cell regularity. The early stage of development of the fertilized egg is called an embryo.

If you remember from high school biology one sperm

fertilizes the egg using enzymes from the sperm head (acrosome). Once in the egg, the egg's cell membrane changes so that no other sperm can penetrate it. Once the egg is fertilized it starts to divide and the division of cells is called cleavage. This occurs in the early development of the embryo.

What are the criteria the embryologist is using in grading the embryos?

Once fertilization has occurred, the embryologist look for the following:

1) Cell number: Normal development of the embryos should be at two to four cells by 48 hours after egg retrieval; at day three the embryo should have eight cells.

2) Cell regularity or symmetry: The divided cells should all be about the same size or symmetrical.

3) Cell fragmentation: This is when parts of the individual cells in the embryo break apart or fragment and appear as small fragments or blebs in the embryo. In some cases the amount of fragmentation is related to the overall quality of the embryo. Embryos with extensive fragmentation have been known to have lower implantation results.[135]

"The ASRM (American Society for Reproductive Medicine) has attempted to establish a standard grading system, so when a patient or previous clinic is talking about 'the quality of the embryos', it can be interpreted and understood by the clinic she is now at, which is important in trying to understand why her cycle of IVF was unsuccessful and what 'changes' can be made to result in a successful outcome. Even with a standardized grading system, which is still not universally used, evaluation and scoring of any stage of embryo development, from fertilization to hatching blastocyst is critical to the experience and expertise of the embryologist."[136]

The hatching blastocyst occurs when the embryo breaks through the zona pellucida, which has to happen for the embryo to implant in the uterus. The zona pellucida is a membrane around the egg that binds with the sperm for fertilization to occur. The breakdown of the zona is called hatching.

I'm sure you remember in school that getting an A on a quiz was better than a B and a B was better than a C. When it comes to "grading," what does the grade mean in terms of embryos development? The answer is not a simple one. The grading system is merely a tool used by the RE and embryologist to determine on what day to transfer and the appropriate number of embryos to transfer back into the uterus -- along with other criteria such as the age of the patient, fertility history and other information. A poor grade does not mean that the baby will be abnormal. It simply means that the chances of implantation are reduced.

All embryo-grading systems are subjective. Based upon the experience of many embryologists grading millions of embryos, we can make educated guesses about an embryo's potential. Even so, there are many cases in which embryos with poor grades result in pregnancies, while others with perfect embryos does not. No matter the grading system, embryo grades do not measure the development inside the embryo genetically.

The fertilization process is a very complicated process and there are many variables involved. Poor results can be devastating to patients and, depending upon preliminary results and in spite of everyone's good efforts, there might still be poor results. Patients with poor fertilization results may move on to (Intracytoplasmic sperm Injection) ICSI on the next cycle, thus taking natural fertilization out of the picture. Complete failure of fertilization occurs much less with ICSI then just plain IVF, but it can still occur.

Once the sperm is inside of the egg complicating issues can still arise. The genetic material of the sperm (the male pronucleus) and the genetic material of the egg (the female pronucleus) fuse to form an embryo. Yet sometimes the egg or sperm do not form the pronucleus, making it impossible to fuse the two together. This results in fertilization failure.

Have I lost you yet?

Sometimes more than one sperm fertilizes an egg. That embryo would not be transferred back because of chance of there being too many chromosomes, which would affect proper development. Or, sometimes the fertilized egg breaks down and stops dividing, which also results in low fertilization results.

I can remember a patient telling me she had a good number of eggs and her husband had a good sperm count. Nevertheless, not one egg fertilized in an IVF cycle. This was one of the few couples I can remember that were unable to get pregnant. The whole process of creating a child under "normal" conditions is quite a miracle. And now, with performing IVF, it is still a miracle by recreating the whole wonderful process outside the body.

IVF labs may assess the embryos at day three or day five (the latter being the blastocyst stage). Each IVF lab has its own protocols for determining when to grade, depending upon the number of embryos and if they are of high enough quality to allow them to make it to the blastocyst stage. A blastocyst is the final stage of the embryo's development before it hatches out of its shell (zona pellucida) and implants in the uterus. The embryos that go to day five have a better success rate and less chance for multiple births.

The goal of the IVF and embryo cultures is to produce high quality embryos. With the improvement of embryo media some labs have better success of reaching the day-5 blastocyst stage. Remember there are so many variables that could affect reaching that stage. So some labs still perform the transfers on day three with success.

How many embryos do you transfer?

Each IVF lab has its own protocols. Depending upon the fertilization results, the patient will come back on either day three or day five following the retrieval date. The numbers of embryos transferred depends upon how many embryos have formed and grades ascribed to them. Other factors also come into play, including the patient's age and past fertility history. Also, there is an increasing focus upon elective single embryo transfer (eSET) so as to reduce the risk of multiple pregnancies.

These factors likewise influence the pregnancy rate and multiple pregnancy rates. Statistics show higher success rates for implantation after embryo transfer in younger patients. For example if you are in your twenties or early thirties and, through IVF, have transferred back two embryos, chances are good that the patient may have twins. In older patients, the RE may place back more than two embryos since chances of failure to implant will be higher. (Even so it remains possible that multiple births can occur.)[137]

Each center looks at each recipient's medical history and individual circumstances to determine the right course. (For example, if the procedure is the last IVF cycle this patient will undergo, the specialist may consider adding one more embryo.)

Mary's eggs had been in a petri dish with Tim's sperm for two days. The nurse checked her fertilization results and called her saying she had five embryos in total, and three embryos graded as a "3" ("4" being the best grade for this clinic). Mary is told she doesn't have enough embryos to go to the blastocyst stage and that she will do her transfer on day three.

If a patient has a high number of embryos with high grades they may be able to freeze some and save them for a future cycles (called "frozen" cycles).[138] The embryos must be of high quality to be frozen because they undergo the additional step of thawing before they can be used. Every step introduces the possibility of change in the outside cell membrane, which can lessen the chance for successful implantation. The RE will talk to Mary and Tim and decide how many embryos to transfer into Mary's uterus. In Mary's case she did not have enough to freeze.

Mary and Tim signed a consent form before the IVF procedure. They made the decision that, if there are any embryos left over that will not be used, the couple has a choice of disposing of them or donating them to research. Donating them would help in training the lab staff on techniques for ICSI and Assisted Hatching. In this case, Mary and Tim chose to donate the extra embryos to research.

Assisted Hatching[139]

Assisted hatching is a relatively new technique used during certain IVF procedures. It is performed to help an embryo "hatch out" of its protective layering and implant into the uterus. This is done for patients who have had failed previous IVF cycles. (This may be due to the embryo not hatching on its own from the zona pellucida or if a women is over 37 years of age or possesses a high Day-3 FSH level.)

The zona pellucida (ZP), as noted, is the protective covering of proteins that surrounds embryo until it reaches Day-5 blastocyst stage. At this point it needs to hatch out from the ZP so it can implant in the uterine lining. Sometimes the embryo has a hard time hatching from the ZP because the covering can be too thick or the embryo doesn't have enough energy to break through. Assisted Hatching is performed a few hours before the transfer under the microscope by means of a poking a small hole in the ZP through which a small amount of acid buffer is introduced. The acid breaks down the outer lining of the ZP and the embryos are then washed in another solution and placed back in the incubator. The embryos will be transferred into to the uterus one to three hours from performing the Assisted Hatching.

What Should Mary Expect on Transfer Day?

The actual transfer is a simple procedure much like a pap smear or an IUI. The exception is that the patient will need a full bladder for the transfer. The embryo(s) are placed in a catheter and then inserted into the uterus. The RE and embryologist will confirm the name and date-of-birth of the recipient to make sure it matches the embryo(s). The procedure takes place in a sterile setting but the recipient will not be put under sedation. The embryos are transferred into a catheter and a speculum is placed in the female. Ultra sound guidance may be used to help guide the catheter and confirm placement in the uterus. This is the point where the previous mock transfer aids in the process. The RE is already aware of potential difficulties in the transfer.

The embryo transfer technique is an important variable in the procedure. A smooth transfer with no trauma to the endometrial lining is essential to give the embryos the best chance for implantation. The embryo(s) are transferred in the uterus and hopefully will implant. The RE will pass the catheter back to the embryologist to flush the catheter and look under the scope to be sure all embryo(s) were transferred. There should be very little pain during the transfer, though it may cause mild cramping. There is a small risk of bleeding or infection.

What Next?

After transfer a brief recovery period Mary will get dressed and leave. Her doctor may require strict bed rest or she may be asked to limit sexual activities and taking baths. On these matters and other questions she may possess, she will be sure to double check with her RE and her nurse.

Implantation can occur two to four days after the transfer. Mary should continue all medications that have been prescribed to her by the RE. A pregnancy test will be given 14 days after the transfer, regardless of the presence of any uterine bleeding. Patients have told me that the 14-day waiting period[140] is the hardest part of the IVF cycle. The patient is wondering constantly: Did it work? Am I pregnant?

Mary will return to the clinic to have blood drawn for a pregnancy test on the 14th day after the transfer. She is told not to do a home pregnancy test because the HCG shot she took to facilitate ovulation is also the hormone that identifies pregnancy. Trace amount of HCG from the previous injection may remain in her body, which could render a false positive. Even if she experiences spotting or feels like she is getting her period, Mary still will come in for the blood test. (Sometimes women may have more than one embryo and one might not have implanted which may cause the spotting or bleeding.)

When the embryo(s) implant in the uterus, let's say around day four, the embryo then starts producing the pregnancy hormone - Human Chorionic Gonadotropin (HCG). This is what is measured in a standard blood pregnancy test. You will have an HCG test drawn and the RE likes to see the HCG result around 150 mIU/ml (milli-international units). It is possible the number could be less and this could be due to an embryo implanting a day later. The patient then returns in 48 hours for a second pregnancy test and the number should have doubled to 300, which shows a good pregnancy.[141]

The nurse will be excited to call Mary and tell her the pregnancy test registered positive, with a quantitative HCG count at 250. The nurse answers further questions that Mary may ask and confirms that she is taking prenatal vitamins (or checks to see if she needs a prescription for them). (Most patients will have started taking a good multiple vitamins with folic acid while trying to get pregnant.) She then instructs Mary to return in two days for follow-up test, which should have a count of 600. At the time of the second blood test (48 hours following the positive pregnancy result) the nurse booked an ultrasound to take place two weeks following that date. The ultrasound will indicate how many embryos successfully implanted.[142]

Before the transfer, Mary and Tim had decided to have two embryos transferred back. The ultrasound now indicates that they were pregnant with twins. They were excited and had many questions for the specialist. The specialist reviews their questions and wants to confirm that Mary has an OB-GYN picked out for further care during the developing pregnancy. Needless to say she expressed profound gratitude to the doctor and staff for the wonderful treatment she and Tim received.

Not everyone's result has the same satisfactory ending,

however. There are many instances when the couple does not succeed in getting pregnant during their first IVF cycle. Let's say Mary did not get pregnant after the first cycle. She would be instructed to stop taking the progesterone and expect to get her period within two to five days. (In the event she did not start her period after five days she would contact her nurse.) It is helpful to set up a follow-up consult with the specialist within a few weeks after the HCG results. It is very important to talk about what's next.

The specialists would review the previous cycle, looking at medications, the number of eggs produced, sperm counts, and fertilization results. Then they will determine what, if anything should be changed or adjusted for the upcoming cycle. If the follicle numbers were low they may switch medications or do a flare protocol. If the fertilization results were low or sperm motility was low, they may try an ICSI cycle wherein the sperm is injected in the egg.

For those patients who are on their third IVF cycle and still not pregnant, the RE may suggest Assisted Hatching on the next cycle (discussed above), which helps with implantation. Another IVF cycle could start as soon as the next month after a failed cycle. These special procedures cost more money than the standard IVF procedure and may not be covered by insurance companies.

Some patients choose take a break for a few months to allow their bodies recover. This may be a good time to talk with the counselor or join a support group. It is also a great time to consider relaxation therapies, such as a massage, a Reiki treatment, or acupuncture.

Preimplantation Genetic Diagnosis (PGD)[143]

Preimplantation Genetic Diagnosis (PGD) is a new advanced reproductive technology used in conjunction with IVF for diagnosis of genetic disease in the embryo(s) before transferring them back to the patient. It is being used widely in most IVF centers and has increased the success rates for an IVF pregnancy in couples that have had previous IVF failures.

Embryologists grade the embryos on day three after retrieval. They look at their fertilization results (meaning the number of eggs fertilized) and document on your records the results based upon the quality of the embryo according to its cell number, cell regularity or symmetry and cell fragmentation. The advanced nature of PGD technology has shown that an embryo that might otherwise have been graded as poor quality was actually genetically normal and therefore could produce a normal pregnancy. (Before PGD this embryo would not have been selected for transfer.) The opposite is also true. An embryo might have been graded as being of good quality and would be selected for transfer, without knowing it actually possessed some genetic abnormalities and would end in a miscarriage.

PGD has given a new tool for physicians to examine the embryo beyond the appearance to being able to read its genetic code. The test takes one or two cells out of a day-three embryo(s) and tests the cells for the genetic makeup by looking at the chromosomes of the embryo. In humans each cell normally contains 23 pairs of chromosomes for a total of 46. Twenty-two of the pairs look the same in a male or female but the 23rd pair is the sex chromosome, which distinguishes between a male and female. The female has two copies of the X chromosome (XX) and the male has an X and Y chromosome (XY). Chromosomes that result in an abnormal embryo may not implant and be miscarried. PGD allows the embryologists to separate normal from abnormal embryos. The normal embryos will be transferred back to the patient. This has improved the success for IVF.

Some reasons why couples consider PGD include: failed IVF cycles because of recurrent miscarriages; maternal age over 35 years; a child or family history of genetic abnormalities (such as Cystic Fibrosis); polycystic ovary syndrome (PCOS); and premature ovarian failure.

Risk of chromosomal abnormalities in pregnancy increases precipitously in women with after they've reached the age of 35. At this age there is also a higher risk of having a child with Down syndrome, called Trisomy 21. A woman's age also affects the possibility of aneuploidy, a condition that occurs when there exists an abnormal number of chromosomes (an extra or missing chromosome), which causes genetic disorders (birth defects).

The accuracy of PGD in determining genetic abnormalities exceeds 98 percent.[144] Once the genetic information is known for each embryo the RE sits down with the couple to discuss the health of each embryo. The couple, knowing this information, diminishes the number of embryos transferred back, decreasing multiple births and premature pregnancies, while optimizing the possibility of success. This also allows for freezing the extra normal embryos for future pregnancies.[145]

Using PGD to select the best embryos is clearly superior to methods of selection. Miscarriage rates following PGD are far less then those in a standard IVF cycle.

Further, if the results of PGD determine that despite all medical intervention, a couple still is unable to have a healthy pregnancy, then it enables them come to terms with their infertility and have peace in the knowledge that they tried everything possible. (If this is the case, some opt to go to the next step of using donor eggs, to be discussed in Chapter 22.)

PGD is a significant scientific advancement in the science of IVF and has helped to explain IVF failure while increasing success rates for couples.

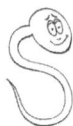

Spanky says:

"A patient is having an IUI and her husband says:
'I'm a really good swimmer and
couldn't get those across the finish line.
I hope the nurse has a better shot than I.'"

Chapter 19
Risks & Complications of IVF Treatment & Procedures

Inevitably there are risk factors associated with IVF. These include:

- Multiple births
- Ovarian hyperstimulation syndrome (OHSS)
- Miscarriages
- Risks Associated with ICSI
- Risks Associated with Assisted Hatching
- Ectopic pregnancy (Tubal Pregnancy)
- Molar pregnancy
- Fertility Drugs and Ovarian Cancer

Multiple Births

"Multiple pregnancy and births are the most common and most serious complications of assisted reproductive technology. Multiple births are associated with higher rates of preterm delivery, low birth weight, congenital anomalies, infant death, and disability among survivors. Carrying a multiple gestation pregnancy is associated with adverse maternal outcomes, such as hemorrhage, pregnancy-induced hypertension and anemia, as well as maternal mortality. The rate of multiple births in the USA has increased markedly during the past two decades largely due to the increased use of fertility treatments, including assisted reproductive technology. Transferring multiple embryos in order to increase the chance of pregnancy and live birth is a common practice among assisted reproductive technology providers, and it results in a high proportion of multiples among assisted reproduction-conceived infants."[146]

The recent success of the culture media for the embryos to go to the day-5 blastocyst stage allows for selection of the best quality of embryos for the transfer. Embryo quality is very important for a successful IVF cycle. The five-day transfer means fewer embryos need to be transferred, which reduces the risk of multiple births while maintaining high IVF success rates.[147]

However, it has been identified that there is an increased possibility of having monozygote twins[148] in patients undergoing ART procedures, including IVF and ICSI. Identified risks include age of the patient, treatment regimen (stimulation of ovaries), and micromanipulation of the embryo during ICSI and Assisted Hatching. To perform ICSI and Assisted Hatching the embryologists use a special microscope that has the necessary tools that enable them to inject the egg with the sperm (ICSI) or put a small hole in the side of the embryo (Assisted Hatching). This type of tool that attaches to a microscope is called a micromanipulator. This handling of the egg and embryo could cause the splitting of an egg into two. Blastocyst transfer has also shown an increase of monozygote twins. This occurs when some time after five days the egg splits into two on its own. In some cases this is less than one percent, meaning it is rare. But it can happen. So if two embryos are transferred and they are successful in implantation and then one splits on its own, the patient would give birth to triplets. Researchers are evaluating this and trying to understand more specifically why this occurs and to see if something can be done to lower the numbers for monozygote twins.[149]

During the IVF cycle, when the ovaries are stimulated to produce as many eggs as possible, the patient is instructed by the nurse to refrain from intercourse a certain number of days prior to the retrieval day (especially if she still has her own fallopian tubes and her partner doesn't possess a male factor). Some also include the time when the patient is on FSH medications to produce multiple eggs. There is a chance that an egg(s) could be tucked up in an area that might be missed during retrieval. If she had intercourse, after which the sperm stays alive for a few days, she might get pregnant on her own along with the two embryos that will be placed back in on transfer day. This is called Concurrent IVF Spontaneous Conception. There are not too many times that you are told not to have intercourse during your treatment, but this one is important.[150]

Ovarian Hyperstimulation Syndrome (OHSS)
Anytime a patient takes medication, possible side effects or complications can occur, and some people are

more susceptible than others. OHSS is a serious complication in IVF. It can happen during the follicle-stimulating phase of a fertility therapy (FSH injections) but it usually occurs when you receive the injection of HCG to trigger ovulation. Typically, signs and symptoms appear within the first 10 days after the injection when the ovarian blood vessels have an abnormal reaction to the hormone and begin to leak fluid. This fluid can swell the ovaries and sometimes moves into the abdomen in large amounts.

There are two types of OHSS: Early-onset OHSS, which develops after the pre-retrieval HCG injection; and late-onset OHSS, which develop when the treatment is successful and pregnancy follows. If the treatment does not lead to pregnancy, early-onset OHSS usually resolves on its own within a few days. It can result in some ovarian enlargement with slight abdominal pain, swelling due to a minimal amount of fluid in the abdomen. The standard medical treatment is pain relief and bed rest and the symptoms will go away. The body will reabsorb this fluid and the fluid will also be voided (urination) out the body. Late-onset OHSS, on the other hand, can persist for weeks during early pregnancy because the body is producing the pregnancy hormone HCG. Not only did the patient have the injection of HCG, but also if she is pregnant her body is also now producing it. HCG seems to plays an important role in the cause of both types of OHSS.

Ovarian Hyperstimulation Syndrome may be classified as mild, moderate or severe depending upon the symptoms. The worst cases tend to be associated with pregnancy. Severe OHSS is a life threatening complication following ovarian stimulation.

Very rarely the ovarian hyperstimulation is severe and the ovaries are very swollen. The patient will feel ill, with nausea and vomiting, abdominal pain. Fluid accumulates in the abdominal cavity and chest, causing abdominal swelling and shortness of breath. Reduction in the amount of urine produced. These complications require urgent hospital admission to restore the fluid and electrolyte balance, monitor progress, control pain and in some very serious cases, include the termination of the pregnancy. Complications associated with severe OHSS include blood-clotting disorders, kidney damage and twisted ovary (ovarian torsion).

The majority of women have a mild or moderate form of the syndrome and invariably it resolves within a few days unless pregnancy occurs, which may delay recovery. The patient may complain of pain or may have a bloated feeling and mild abdominal swelling. For a small number of women the degree of discomfort can be quite pronounced. The severity is graded on the size of the ovaries, subjective complaints, and laboratory/radiologic findings.[151]

If the patient experiences any of the symptoms she must call her specialist as soon as possible. She will then be called in for an ultrasound and blood work. Depending on the severity she might be sent home and told to rest, or she may be admitted to the hospital. It is important to differentiate between OHSS and other conditions that can present in a similar manner. These include ovarian torsion, hemorrhage and pelvic infection following egg collection, ectopic pregnancy and appendicitis.

Incidence of OHSS

Despite careful monitoring, up to 33 percent of IVF treatments have been reported to be associated with mild forms of OHSS. Severe OHSS has been reported in three to eight percent of IVF cycles.[152]

Causes of OHSS [153]

The primary cause of OHSS is a patient's over-response to fertility drugs. Why they have this over-response is unknown. Women at risk of developing OHSS include:

- Young thin women (< 30 yrs)
- High estrogen hormone levels and a large number of follicles or eggs.
- Administration of medication that prevents ovulation (Lupron)
- The use of HCG for luteal phase support.
- Past history of OHSS

Patient Instructions[154]

- Weigh yourself daily - starting on the first day you begin injections
- Drink plenty of fluids. Fluids with electrolytes and salts such as Gatorade and V8 are best. Avoid ONLY drinking plain water. Be sure to drink at least one liter of fluid daily. Eat salty snacks such as pret-

zels and potato chips.

- Monitor your urine. Dark urine signals dehydration. Be sure to drink enough fluid to keep your urine a light color. Please let us know if you notice a significant decrease in the amount of urine you void.
- Periodically stretch your legs and wiggle your toes.
- Pelvic rest; no intercourse, tampons, pelvic Ultrasound or examinations. If you must be seen in an Emergency Room, DO NOT allow anyone to do a bimanual pelvic exam. (This is where the physician does a pelvic exam placing a finger inside the vagina and a placing other hand on the lower part of the abdomen)
- Limit lifting to 5 pounds.
- Avoid constipation; drink fluids; eat raw fruits; vegetables and high fiber cereals.

What is the treatment of OHSS?

There is no specific treatment for OHSS. Therapy is based on supportive care until the condition resolves spontaneously. Treatment is guided by the severity of OHSS. Women with mild OHSS and some women with moderate OHSS can be managed on an outpatient basis. Women with severe OHSS and some women with moderated OHSS require admission to the hospital. The aim of the treatment is to help relieving symptoms and prevent complications.

Those at risk need to be identified and an appropriate stimulation protocol needs to be chosen. If the patient still hyper-responds, the dose of medication can be reduced or withheld during stimulation; or embryos can be frozen instead of being transferred and the cycle can be canceled.[155]

Miscarriages

Miscarriage is perhaps the most difficult medical event that some couples must deal with. It is especially stressful and traumatic if the couple conceived using advanced reproductive technologies such as IVF. There is a profound sense of loss coupled with the emotional and financial stresses that accompany these therapies. It is true that some research shows that pregnancies conceived via IVF carry a slightly increased risk of miscarriage compared to spontaneous pregnancies. The exact level of the increased risk varies by study.[156]

Most researchers believe that the increased risks for miscarriages is not related to the IVF procedure itself, but related more to the underlying reasons for infertility treatment. Reasons for miscarriages can range from the partners ages that affect the quality of the eggs and sperm, to problems with the uterus, hormonal imbalances, fibroids, and chromosome abnormalities. These are the most plausible explanations as determined from studies, and they are not related to IVF procedure.

One study in Denmark showed an increase in miscarriage rate with advanced maternal age is caused by a decline in oocyte quality (immature eggs). These patients showed a poor response to the hyperstimulation of the ovaries and produced very few eggs. The study compared women who were under the age of 36 and looked

at miscarriage rates between normal and poor responders to hyperstimulation of the ovaries and saw no difference. But there was a significant increased rate of miscarriage for women over 36 years of age.[157]

We had a case in which a patient having multiple miscarriages. Tests determined that a large percentage of
the partner's sperm possessed a genetic abnormality
that caused miscarriage. Researchers looking further into
failed IUI and IVF cycles looked at the DNA of the sperm
and found that many infertile men have a high DNA
Fragmentation Index (DFI).[158]

There is a group of blood tests that the RE will check
which looks at the genetic makeup of both partners and
look into antibodies in the blood of the female. Others
may have a reason that is not so easy to address. Regardless, if IVF is a treatment the patient desires to explore
seriously, she ought to follow through and work with the
specialist despite these risks and contingencies.[159]

Risks associated with ICSI

The ICSI procedure has helped many families to have
their own children with the male partner having male
factor (low sperm count, low motility and abnormal morphology of sperm). Male factor can be associated with
in some cases chromosomal abnormalities and genetic
abnormalities. In 20 percent of the male with male factor has some form of "Y micro deletion" where the "Y"
chromosome is missing or has missing genes. Let's keep
in mind that in normal conception these sperm wouldn't
normally fertilize the egg, but with ICSI the eggs are be-

ing fertilized. That being said there is a risk of having a child with chromosomal abnormality.

Another risk factor is during the ICSI procedure a small number of eggs—usually less than five percent—can be damaged as a result of the needle insertion.

It is important to understand that the following problems can be associated with sex chromosome abnormalities:[160]

- Increased risk of miscarriage
- Heart problems for affected infants that may require surgery
- Increased risk of behavior or learning disabilities
- Increased risk of infertility in your children during their adulthood

Several studies have addressed the issue of developmental delays in children born of ICSI. However, there is no conclusive evidence that this is the case.

It is recommended that patients who get pregnant after an ICSI procedure seek prenatal testing either by means of an amniocentesis (taking a sample of amniotic fluid) or a chronic villus sampling (biopsy of the uterus) to check for fetal abnormalities. Also, patients should have a level II ultrasound, which is usually performed around 16 weeks gestation. The safety and success of ICSI is still being looked at closely. It remains a new technique with uncertainty about all of the outcomes. Selection of the most normal looking sperm does not ensure that the sperm is normal.[161]

Risks associated with Assisted Hatching

Unfortunately, there are some risks associated with Assisted Hatching procedures as well. In particular, Assisted Hatching procedures seem to increase the likelihood that you will have identical twins (also known as monozygote twins). This is because the micromanipulation technique used to break through the zona pellucida can sometimes cause the embryo to split into two identical halves. There is also an increased risk of:

- damage to the embryo, potentially causing death
- fetal complications
- physical deformity
- conjoined twins

The mother is put on steroids and antibiotics to help decrease the possibility of the body rejecting the embryo. The steroids have their own side effects like: high blood pressure, infection, nausea and mood swings. [162]

It is recommended that patients who get pregnant after Assisted Hatching procedure seek prenatal testing either getting an amniocentesis or a chronic villus sampling to check for any fetal abnormalities, along with a level II ultrasound that is usually performed around 16 weeks of gestation. Like ICSI, the safety and success of AH is still being looked at closely, being considered a new technique without knowing all the outcomes.

IVF and Ectopic Pregnancy[163]

One of the potential risks of fertility treatments such

as IVF and IUI is the increased chance of ectopic pregnancy. Ectopic pregnancy occurs when a woman's egg is fertilized by her partner's sperm and the resulting embryo implants somewhere outside the woman's uterus. An embryo that is growing outside the uterus creates a potentially life-threatening situation for both mother and the fetus. Although ectopic pregnancies can occur also when a woman conceives naturally, fertility treatments such as IVF or IUI increase a patient's chances that her pregnancy might be ectopic.[164]

How Does this Happen?

During a normal pregnancy, a sperm inside the fallopian tubes fertilizes an egg. The fertilized egg travels down the fallopian tubes to the uterus, where it implants on the inside wall and will grow into a healthy baby over the next nine months. An ectopic pregnancy occurs when the fertilized egg implants outside the uterus -- in most cases, in the fallopian tubes, which is called a tubal pregnancy. There are some rare cases where the fertilized egg can implant on an ovary, within a cervix or abdomen. The danger associated with this is that the affected organ can rupture and cause severe bleeding. When this occurs the embryo cannot survive and an ectopic can be very dangerous for the mother if not treated.

IVF Transfer

During IVF treatment the eggs are removed from the mother and placed in petri dish along with her partner's sperm. During the transfer the embryos are injected into the uterus. Nevertheless it is possible that they can be inadvertently injected too high up in the uterus or the specialist injects them with such force that the embryos can end up floating around and possibly implanting themselves in places where they shouldn't. There is also a chance of an ectopic pregnancy with an IUI procedure, even though the sperm is injected in the uterus but fertilization still occurs in the fallopian tubes.

What Are The Chances?

There is a two-to-five percent chance of IVF treatments ending in an ectopic pregnancy. If the patient is undergoing either IVF or IUI treatment and she does get pregnant, she and her specialist must be vigilant about possible symptoms of an ectopic pregnancy. [165]

Ectopic Pregnancy Symptoms

If you have any of the following symptoms let your nurse and RE know as soon as possible.

Initially an ectopic pregnancy may appear as a normal pregnancy with a missed period, sore breasts and nausea. However there is often abnormal vaginal bleeding after expected period and pain on the side of the tube affected and you may experience light-headedness. If the tube ruptures this results in severe abdominal pain, fainting and shock. Some women (approximately 50 percent) have no symptoms until the tube ruptures. Diagnosis of the ectopic was usually made after the tube ruptured and the patient was rushed to the emergency room. Ectopic pregnancies rarely resolve on their own and can pose a risk to the mother. So early detection and treatment is better for everyone.[166]

How is an Ectopic diagnosed?

The good news is that today an ectopic can be diagnosed early by means of a blood test and measuring the HCG level, along with a vaginal ultrasound. Both tests are performed together in order to interpret them correctly. Beta HCG is a very specific hormone marker for pregnancy. This blood test is very sensitive and if it is negative, can exclude any risk for a significant ectopic pregnancy. A positive HCG level confirms the patient is pregnant, but does not tell us where the embryo is located. A normal HCG level doubles in number over a 48-hour period. This is why the RE will have you come in for the initial HCG blood test and return two days later for another blood sample. The RE wants to see the HCG level double in number from the first blood draw. Low or slowing increasing levels of HCG could suggest and problem pregnancy and, in this case, the RE will request that an ultrasound be performed. If the ultrasound shows no pregnancy, than an ectopic is suspected. Sometimes it is difficult to distinguish between an ectopic and an early miscarriage. A laparoscopy could confirm the diagnosis, which will show a pregnancy in the tube.[167]

How is an Ectopic treated?

The major benefit of early diagnosis is that early treatment can save the fallopian tube, thus preserving fertility for the future.

Ectopics are being treated with an anti-cancer drug called Methotrexate, an intramuscular shot that kills the rapidly growing dividing cells of the tubal pregnancy.

The RE wants to see HCG levels at zero, so this means the patient will be returning for several blood draws. (She must remember to drink water before hand!) Depending on how quickly the HCG level is dropping, the patient may get more injections of medication. Methotrexate injections can replace surgery as long as the HCG level is dropping. Your RE will be watching very closely during this critical time. A zero result confirms the pregnancy has been destroyed successfully.

Surgical treatment can be done if diagnosed early through a laparoscope as well with salpingostomy. The pregnancy can be removed and the tube can be saved. A salpingostomy is the formation of an artificial opening in a fallopian tube to restore itself to normal in the event that the opening was blocked closed by an infection or chronic inflammation.

Women with moderate or strong risk factors for ectopic pregnancy, and those who conceived after IVF, are often monitored with ultrasound and blood testing after their first missed period to detect and treat a potential ectopic pregnancy.

If a tube ruptures and blood collects in the abdomen, emergency surgery needs to be performed. In these cases the tube needs to be removed because it is so badly damaged because of previous ectopic or a large tubal pregnancy. This is needed to control bleeding. When this occurs the couple mourns the loss of a pregnancy along with losing a fallopian tube.[168]

How does an ectopic pregnancy affect future fertility?

Sometimes tubal pregnancy can affect both sides of the fallopian tubes, which increases the chance of being perpetually infertile because of the possibility of both tubes rupturing and the need to be removed. In the case of not having any fallopian tubes your RE would move you right to IVF treatment, because IVF bypasses the tubes to begin with. The risk of having a repeat ectopic is increased even if the other tube seems normal. However, 60 percent of women who have had a tubal pregnancy the first time will have a normal pregnancy the next time without further treatment. Early testing is the key to rule out an ectopic pregnancy. In general, women can have an ectopic pregnancy with natural conception and not be in an infertility program.

Having an unsuccessful outcome the first time can be very stressful and discouraging. But with the right treatment there is a very good chance of having a baby. Remember having an ectopic shows the sperm and egg are good.[169]

Molar Pregnancy

Abnormal pregnancies, generally, are surprisingly common and can happen to any woman. A molar pregnancy is one of those abnormalities and can have extreme side effects that can damage the body. A molar pregnancy is also called Gestational Trophoblastic Disease (GTD) and a hydatidiform mole. A molar pregnancy occurs when a genetic error occurs during fertilization and causes an abnormal growth in the uterus.

There are two types of molar pregnancy: complete and partial. A complete molar pregnancy occurs when a sperm fertilizes a nonviable egg resulting in the growth of an abnormal placenta. The placenta grows and in turn produces very high level of HCG. A partial molar pregnancy occurs when two sperm fertilize one egg and the embryo does not survive (having an extra 23 chromosomes). During these types of pregnancies the placenta produces abnormal sacs, which resemble grapes.[170]

Signs and Symptoms

The signs of a molar are very similar to a regular pregnancy: a missed period and morning sickness. As the pregnancy progresses other symptoms may appear, such as vaginal bleeding, severe nausea, no fetal heartbeat, high HCG levels and an expanding uterus.

The risk of molar pregnancy is increased in women over the age of 35; in women who have previously had a molar pregnancy; and in women with a history of miscarriages.[171]

How is a Molar diagnosed?

A molar pregnancy is diagnosed by a pelvic exam, ultrasound and HCG blood draws. Being in an infertility program the patient is being closely monitored with blood work and ultrasounds. When the RE first learns that a patient is pregnant by a positive HCG level, she

279

will have a second HCG level two days later, along with an ultrasound two weeks after that. A molar pregnancy produces such high HCG levels that the RE picks up on this right away. A molar pregnancy is confirmed when the first ultrasound does not show a fetus.[172] The ultrasound will show the placenta as a cluster of grapes.

How are Molar pregnancy treated?

Sometimes a molar pregnancy will spontaneously end and the patient will expel a tissue that looks like a grape. If it doesn't expel on its own, the mole needs to be removed and it will be removed by a D & C (dilation and curettage). The RE will have the patient continue with the blood draws to check HCG levels until the number registers negative. (Sometimes there is a piece of tissue left that could be producing HCG and it takes a while for the HCG to become negative. Women wonder why it takes so long to get a negative result because they may come in weekly for the blood draw and it could take a couple of months.) Women who have had a molar pregnancy can be at risk of having another. The doctor will watch her closely and may have her use contraception for a while to prevent pregnancy; most physicians want the patient to take a year off of fertility treatments.

In most cases GTDs are benign and not cancerous. In rare cases some may malignant (which means cancerous). This type of cancer is usually very easy to treat and has a high percentage rate for curing it.[173]

Women who suffer with this type of abnormal pregnancy may fall into depression. Even though a real baby is not in this pregnancy, women feel as if the failure is their fault. Added to this, the body has produced all kinds of hormones. These symptoms can also resemble postpartum depression – when a woman goes into a deep depression after having a child or being pregnant. These feelings can be normal. Even so, women should seek mental health care and, if necessary, treatment.

After the mole is removed, most women abstain from getting pregnant for a while. It is preferable to wait about a year. The longer between pregnancies the higher chance for a successful pregnancy.[174]

Fertility Drugs and Cancer Risk [175]

All medications, including infertility drugs come with risks. With the field of infertility ever expanding and, thus with the increase of the use of medications such as Clomid (and hyperstimulation drugs), physicians and patients are concerned about the possible cancer risks associated with these medications. I have researched this, reading articles and studies that seek to determine if there is a connection between fertility medication and cancer risks, particularly ovarian, uterine and breast cancer. Fortunately, to date the consensus is that the risk of cancer from the use of these medications (gonadotropins and Clomid) is very low.

It was announced in the recent annual meeting in June 2014 of the European Society of Human Reproduction and Embryology (ESHRE) that research has shown that the use of fertility drugs does not appear to show an increase in breast and gynecological cancers.

Fertility drugs stimulate the ovaries for production of eggs and aid in ovulation, they contain levels of estrogen and progesterone yet their affects on breast and gynecological cancers remain uncertain. Most previous studies of fertility drugs involved small number of patients and the inability to control other cancer predictors where patients can be on other medications that can have increase cancer risks.

In a large 30-year follow-up study, infertility patients from 1965 to1988 at five United States sites and were evaluated. The data was collected through patient questionnaires and links with National Death Index and Cancer registries. The study followed 9,892 women successfully for cancer outcomes. The study revealed, 749 cases of breast cancer, 119 cases of uterine cancer and 85 cases of ovarian cancer were diagnosed among the women. There were limitations to the study to be able to obtain complete risk factor information, including hysterectomy status.

The study showed if Clomid was ever used, was not associated with breast cancer but higher risks were seen when the use of Clomid (Clomiphene) among women heavily exposed for 12 or more cycles and found higher risks of ovarian cancer was seen among women who have never been pregnant or able to conceive.

Of all the infertility drugs used: Clomid and Gonadotropins, Clomid was the most common drug used in the 1980s.

Gonadotropins use was unrelated to cancer risk; few women (10 percent) were exposed.

The study did not show a strong link between use of fertility drugs and breast or gynecological cancers. However, the association of infertility drugs and cancers should be monitored due to the age of this study population and the increased incidence of these cancers.

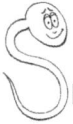

panky says:
*"It is a good time to stop and tell a story.
It is about one of our patients that had
an ectopic and lost a fallopian tube"* ~ ~ ~

Beth first came for infertility help when she was 30 years old. Beth was married for two years and had already had one miscarriage. She and her husband were very anxious to get started. They came to our center a year after we had opened and she just loved her specialist.

Beth started with three IUIs, the first being on Clomid. She got pregnant but miscarried around seven to eight weeks into the pregnancy. Beth took a class on injections and had no problem giving herself the daily injections of FSH. (She couldn't do the big one at the end so her husband did that one.) She underwent two more IUIs, taking the FSH injectables medications.

Not having success in getting pregnant with the IUIs, she and the RE decided to move on to IVF. She did four IVF treatments without success. Beth always produced at least eight to ten eggs with each cycle and had good fertilization results but always did the day-3 transfer, never making it to the day 5-blastocyst stage.

After the fourth failed IVF she talked with the specialist who suggested that she go for a second opinion and suggested another clinic.

Beth went to the recommended clinic where she underwent one IUI, again, without success. So she did one IVF with them and that also failed. The doctor called her to discuss the failed IVF cycle and suggested that she look into donor eggs. Beth was 34 at the time. Beth thought to herself No way! I'm not giving up. Beth felt that going to the new center where she hadn't gotten pregnant, that she was considered a bad statistic for them. She didn't feel the necessary closeness and trust such as she had experieced at the first clinic.

So Beth returned to her original specialist and wanted to "try again."

She consulted again with her favorite specialist, and together they concluded that all her prior female testing (clomid challenge test, hormone levels) looked fine and her husband's semen analysis were also fine. But there was still no answer for why she wasn't getting pregnant. Her specialist wondered if there might some problems at the implantation stage, which could produce a miscarriage. When the embryo implants in the uterus there is an immunologic acceptance between the implanting embryo and the uterus of the mother. If a patient has had recurrent miscarriage (two or more) the RE may order some immunologic blood tests like Antinuclear Antibody, Lupus Anticoagulant and Anticardiolipin antibodies. They had tried assisted hatching but still no success.

Beth heard that acupuncture could help patients with infertility. So she went for a few treatments with the center's acupuncturist. Beth had her sixth IVF, and it worked! Beth was finally pregnant. She felt, that maybe the acupuncture treatment got the blood flowing to her uterus. Beth was pregnant for the first time on her sixth IVF cycle with a little boy.

Shortly after having her first baby boy, Beth was at home on a weekend with her husband and she told him she felt weird and dizzy. They called 911 and Beth found herself in the ER and the doctor asking her: "Do you think you could be pregnant?"

She laughed and said I don't think so, knowing what she has been through. Well the ER discovered that Beth was pregnant and it was a natural pregnancy but it was an ectopic and she had surgery and lost a fallopian tube. She had symptoms but no clue that she was pregnant.

After a period of time she went back to the fertility clinic and wanted to try for another. The specialist said it wouldn't be a problem having only one tube but they would have to do IVF, of course. That particular cycle she had two embryos and bingo she was pregnant and had a little girl (baby number two).

Beth said she could not have gone through this whole ordeal if it wasn't for her support group. She found a forum on-line and connected with some women that were going through the same situations of infertility. Beth said it feels so good to share your story with someone who understands. They all became good friends and still get together a couple of times a year and their children play together.

As the two children started growing, Beth had a yard sale and sold all the baby furniture, clothes and toys. Then, to her surprise – yes! – She was pregnant on her own with child number three. Beth had another son. Who would have thought?

A lot of times patients have their first child as a result of infertility treatment, and then go on to have a couple on their own. We help them get the ball rolling. Beth would say to anyone don't get discouraged, keep plugging.

Chapter 20
Things to Think About

Embryo Freezing

After an embryo transfer some patients will have additional embryos remaining in culture. In this case couples often opt to freeze these embryos, called cryopreservation, for later use. This is possible only with embryos of high quality for the best success rates. If a couple does not conceive with the initial "fresh" cycle, they may use cryopreserved embryos to attempt pregnancy at a lower cost. "Frozen" cycles also pose less health risks to the female since the patient does not take medications to stimulate the ovaries, only those which prepare the uterus for implantation.[176]

As with embryos obtained from a fresh cycle, the implantation success of frozen embryos depends on the age of the woman at the time of retrieval, the stage and grade of the embryo, and the original cause of infertility.[177]

Embryo freezing involves storing viable embryos in sub-zero temperatures for use at a later date (just like storing the sperm and unfertilized eggs, to be discussed in chapters 23 and 24, respectively). Embryos are frozen by vitrification,[178] which is a technique that freezes embryos quickly and is more successful than the slow freeze method previously used.

Cryopreservation is a process to preserve tissues or cells by cooling them to sub-lower temperatures. In treating infertility, sperm, embryos and eggs can all be cryopreserved. These cells contain water to survive and sperm being the smallest of the cells contains less water. When these cells are frozen, a cryoprotectant is added to the samples and this protectant removes the water from the cells. Depending on how soon the water is removed from the cells, there is a chance some of the water could go to crystals because of the low temperature, which can damage the cell structure. This process of cryopreservation is time-sensitive and the results are visualized after the cells are thawed (determining which cells survived the freeze). The process for freezing sperm and embryos using a slow-freeze method has worked. But since the discovery of vitrification, which is a process for quicker freezing of embryos and eggs, this technique has emerged as the best choice for freezing.

Vitrification also uses cryoprotectants, but this technique works faster removing the water from the cells. During vitrification the embryo is frozen one-at-a-time and it is placed in solutions with increased amounts of cryoprotectants. The last step happens in a matter of seconds: the embryo is placed in a very highly concentrated cryoprotectant solution and then quickly put in a straw, which is then sealed and put directly into liquid nitrogen.

A 42-year-old woman became a mother of a healthy boy after having a frozen embryo transfer of an embryo that had been frozen for 20 years. The embryo had come from a couple that had an IVF procedure performed back in 1990 and had extra embryos, which they decided to freeze and donate anonymously. The 42-year-old woman had undergone IVF treatment for 10 years with no success. Twenty years later the extra embryos were offered to her and her husband from a list that offered the best physical match. The couples were aware of the 20-year time period during which the embryos were frozen. Two embryos survived the thaw and both were implanted. One survived and the women had a healthy baby boy. Up to this point the longest known frozen embryo was 13 years.[179]

A study was done in 2008 in which over 11,000 frozen embryos were thawed from IVF patients that had at least one embryo thaw. The study was evaluating the impact of freezing and storage time to embryo survival, implantation ability and pregnancy outcome. Results showed that their cryostorage duration did not have an adverse affect on survival or pregnancy outcome in IVF or egg donation patient.[180]

Cryopreservation puts cells in an unanimated state and as long as the center stores the embryos, eggs or sperm properly, these cells can be stored many years. Keep in mind that the majority of the patients freeze embryos for their own use and will use their embryos up in a short period of time.

When to Cyropreserve?

Women who get early on-set ovarian hyperstimulation syndrome (OHSS) after egg retrieval are prime candidates for cryopreservation, since the cycle had to stop before it could be completed. Ovarian hyperstimulation usually occurs when taking the infertility drugs that stimulate the ovaries to produce eggs. Some women can have a mild or severe case of OHSS and this can occur after egg retrieval, or after egg transfer. If this occurred after egg retrieval your RE would postpone the transfer because the woman is in pain and needs to rest. The embryos from this cycle can be frozen as not to lose them because the transfer is being postponed. The patient would be put at a higher risk if the transfer were to continue because there is a complication in the cycle. By freezing the embryos, we are not wasting a complete cycle; the patient will have a Frozen embryo transfer (FET) once she recovers from the OHSS.

Other women will opt for cryopreservation because they have been diagnosed with cancer. Some cancer treatments will destroy the eggs in a woman's ovary and may leave her sterile. These women can go through IVF, freeze their embryos, receive their cancer treatment. Then, once cured, they use the frozen embryos to attempt pregnancy. (The very same thing is done for men with cancer and they sperm bank before treatment.)[181]

Some IVF labs freeze the embryos on day three or day five. Embryos from the day-5 blastocyst stage have a higher chance of resulting in a live birth, though this does not mean day-three embryos cannot be successful. Embryology looks at the embryos on day three, early in the morning and then gives the recommendation to the doctor. The decision is based on how many embryos have continued to grow and divide on day three as well as quality, if the embryos are to go to day five. Depending on the number and quality of the embryos, the RE will discuss it with the patients and will make an inform decision on whether to freeze or not.

Cryopreservation enables patients to try again using the frozen embryos, which requires less medication and is about a third less expensive than undergoing another fresh cycle. A frozen cycle requires taking only those medications that prepare the uterus for implantation; there is no need to stimulate the ovaries to produce eggs. If the fresh IVF cycle ended up in a pregnancy then she can reserve the frozen embryos for a future family or if it didn't then she can go back next cycle and do a Frozen Embryo Transfer (FET).

Undergoing a frozen cycle also reduces the risk of multiple pregnancies, since patient elects a single embryo transfer (eSET) from a blastocyst-stage embryo, rendering a very good chance of getting pregnant.

The decision about if to freeze, what to freeze and when to freeze require thoughtful consideration before the IVF cycle begins. The patient must keep in mind that the process inevitably confronts the predicament of what to do with the excess embryos. The younger the women are the better chances of producing more eggs, which after fertilization will be embryos. Some patients have numerous unused embryos and it can become a moral and medical dilemma for the clinic and patients if they are viable and yet have no destination. Consent forms (which patients are required to sign before the IVF cycle) exist to address this situation beforehand. The forms indicate that, if the patient opts not to freeze extra embryos, she has the choice to discarding them or donate them for research activities.[182]

There are other considerations to keep in mind before choosing cryopreservation. Patients incur a charge for storing the embryos, and, beyond that, there are no guarantees of getting pregnant; but that said, the improvements using the new freezing technique are improving pregnancy rates. Another matter to consider is the fact that some patients forget about the embryos and many are left abandoned, leaving a difficult situation for the clinic.

Frozen Embryo Dilemma

Let's review the definition of an embryo: The early stages just after fertilization the cell is called a zygote after more development to the blastocyst, which is on day five, this early stage is called an embryo.

When a patient under goes an IVF cycle depending on the age of the patient and how her body reacts to the injectable gonadotropins, a woman can produce a high number of eggs.

These eggs need to be fertilized with the sperm and you need to see your fertilization results. Women between their late 20s and early 30s can produce over 20 eggs in one cycle. Will these all fertilize and have a good grade? A patient from this type of cycle could have a fair amount of embryos to freeze. Women who are older wouldn't produce as many eggs and would have less to freeze. Remember once the eggs are fertilized the RE will transfer back two to three embryos. There is a very good chance that after one IVF cycle there will be embryos to freeze.

What do you do with your unused viable embryos if you feel like your family is complete? The booming fertility business estimates that approximately 20,000 embryos are "leftover," sitting in cold storage.

There are several choices for the biological parents of these embryos: finding a research program or fellow patient to accept a donation; discarding the extra embryos; or doing absolutely nothing (abandoning them). In March 2009 President Obama signed an executive order paving the way for more couples to donate their embryos to stem-cell research.

When a couple begins an IVF cycle they are required to sign many consent forms ahead of time. In part, these forms determine what will be done with frozen embryos and what to do if the couple divorces or passes away during storage. Patients will need to decide what the embryology lab should do with the embryos.

Some clinics will hold on to the embryos for three to five years and then dispose of them (you do sign off on this). If you decide to dispose of the embryos they are disposed in a biohazard container much like when the lab disposes frozen sperm. If you continue to store the embryos, there is a yearly storage fee that would be charged. At the time of signing the consents, some patients say at the initial consult your not really thinking of the embryos until the reality hits and you have embryos.

An article written in the *Boston Globe*[183] discussed the dilemma facing some couples and how it is not an easy decision to make:

"Some patients revise their desires many times before finding resolution they can live with. They struggle with the fact that frozen embryos come from the same physiological elements involved in the IVF cycle from which they bore their children. Some couples feel the deep and painful memory of all they went through to create these embryos and, though they feel their family is complete, feel unable to dispose of the extra embryos. Some also possess religious convictions that make this a very difficult decision."[184]

The article goes on to describe one family who has three children under the age of four. They received a letter from their Infertility clinic inquiring about what to do with her four frozen embryos. The letter gave them 90 days to make a decision. They had the choice of giving them to research, donating them to another infertile couple, dispose of them, or keep them frozen and pay a yearly fee for storage. The family knew their family was complete but has to make a decision, which is not an easy one. No one close to her has ever done this before and she didn't feel right about throwing them away. After careful thought the family decided to give the extra embryos to research to look for a cure of a couple of diseases that ran through their family.[185]

A survey conducted in 2007 by Anne Lyerly of Duke University Medical Center and Ruth Faden of John Hopkins[186] to see how many patients with extra embryos would want to donate them to research. It was discovered that many patients would donate the embryos to research but some desired a "disposal ceremony", in which patients could take their own embryos and dispose of them as they like.

Others wanted a "compassionate transfer," where you talk with your RE and all the embryos would be transferred during a time in your cycle that would not result in a pregnancy. One fertility specialist said the majority of patients do come back to use their embryos but a small group are really trying not to get pregnant again. From the standpoint of the specialist, he would rather not do it that way.[187]

Another family struggled with the decision after having twins and knowing the family was complete. After reviewing all their options and being a Catholic but prochoice they discovered an organization called Nightlight Christian Adoptions of California, since 1997 have offered Invitro patients the chance to choose someone else to adopt their embryos. The wife felt very compelled to be selecting the perspective parents of her embryos. They were looking at 4 couples and found a couple that was a lot like themselves. The embryos were shipped across the country and the new family ended up having a daughter at first and then a son, using all the embryos.

Nightlight Christian adoptions ask the genetic family their preferences for the adoptive families. Couples preferences may be social, financial, religious, how many children in the adoptive family, and the genetic family wants to stay in touch either on their own with adoptive family or through Nightlight. The adoptive family will also give their own preferences and Nightlight will match the preferences from both families and give the information to the genetic family. The genetic family can say yes to the match or pass it on and wait for another adoptive family.

The genetic family gives all their medical history and lab work for infectious disease testing and this will be considered in the adoptive family match.

There is legal paperwork, which needs to be completed by the genetic family and the adoptive family. The paperwork relinquishes the parental rights of the genetic family prior to the embryo transfer to the receiving mother. Once transferred, the embryos belong to adopting parents. At this time everyone involved should know that embryos have a special legal status that is not yet clearly defined. Because of this embryo adoption programs may differ in how they define embryos in their legal agreements. Some may refer to the embryos as a transfer of property while others may use traditional adoptive language into their legal documents. At the time of birth the adoptive parents will be noted as the legal mother and father on birth certificate. [188]

The "Octomom" Situation

Nadya Suleman, also known as the "Octomom," gave birth in 2009 to octuplets (eight babies), becoming the second person in the United States to do so. According to my research, despite conflicting statements about the number of frozen embryos used, Nadya confronted the dilemma about what to do with her many viable embryos, since she didn't want the frozen embryos discarded. She requested that all of the remaining embryos be implanted, despite the norm for women her age (33) to have only two or three. Twelve remaining embryos were transferred resulting in a total of eight live embryos.[189]

The doctor who performed this procedure, Dr. Michael Kamrava, used very poor judgment, as this patient already had six children from other IVF cycles. The board said in the report that Dr. Michael Kamrava committed gross negligence by making "an excess number of embryo transfer" into Nadya. The Medical Board of California voted to revoke his medical license and he was expelled from the American Society for Reproductive Medicine in 2009. This serves as a negative example for the role and judgment of the RE, upon whom the patients depend.[190]

Depending upon age and number of eggs stimulated during IVF, a patient can get quite a few embryos. Remember, embryos will be frozen that have a high grade. If a patient undergoes a couple of frozen cycles, this could use up to two embryos per cycle. So there may be some embryos left over. Patients need to consider this possibility with great earnestness, considering and discussing with the partner about what to do in this case. They must be prepared to ask questions about current research in order to be very clear about what will be done with unclaimed embryos. Religious convictions may overrule certain options.

Frozen Embryo Update

Infertility centers are now seeing with the improvement of vitrification in freezing embryos that there are fewer crystals in the cell, which keeps the outside membrane of the embryo intact. So when they are thawed, they are just like a fresh embryo.[191] In the past before the new technique of vitrification frozen embryos showed less favorable results in pregnancy than fresh embryos. Shady Grove Fertility is seeing about a 95 percent survival rate and there is almost no loss of quality when thawed. Dr Eric Levens says, "Now, those rates of success for frozen embryos are just equal to the rate of using fresh embryos, which opens up a whole new world of possibilities." The possibilities being a FET as mentioned above costs less than a fresh cycle and has less risks factors for the patient.[192]

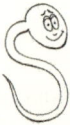

Spanky asked a patient if he was here for an IUI. He said, "Well, I'm not here for a DUI. I need a bigger cup than this!"

Chapter 21
Maternal Fetal Medicine Program

I continue to be amazed at how our society is changing. For example, many people are not wearing watches anymore because they constantly check their cell phones for the time. The sales of newspapers are down since people read the news on the Internet. The United States Post Office is facing lay-offs, since many are paying bills online, using less stamps, and are communicating through email and social media. (Whatever happened to writing letters?)

Keeping pace with the changing world, women are getting pregnant later in life, which comes with its own set of risks. Complicated high-risk pregnancies require optimal care. Patients whose pregnancies fall into this category will go through a program called Maternal Fetal Medicine (MFM).

Woman 35 years or over are considered to be of Advanced Maternal Age (AMA), which puts them in this high-risk category. Women in this category have an increasing possibility of having a child with Down Syndrome, spina bifida and other genetic disorders. Women with medical conditions such as heart disease, diabetes, preeclampsia, genetic disease in the family, and kidney or gastrointestinal disease are also candidates for the MFM protocols. Further, healthy women whose pregnancy carries an increased risk factor because of an abnormal AFP (Alpha Fetoprotein), twins, triplets or more because of preterm labor and recurrent pregnancy loss, premature rupture of membranes, and any other condition from a previous high-risk pregnancy are also candidates for MFM.

Your OB-GYN will set up the appointment where you will have what is called a Level II ultrasound and you'll meet with a genetic counselor to determine if a pregnancy is high-risk. It is very important that both partners attend this appointment since the medical history on both sides of the family will be covered.

Genetic Consultation / Amniocentesis

The first portion of the appointment includes a consultation with a genetic counselor, who reviews and draws a family tree of both families and discusses family history. (It is a good idea to make a list of anything that might be germane, such as, for example, a cousin with Cystic Fibrosis.) The genetic counselor explores the option of having an amniocentesis, a procedure in which amniotic fluid is removed from the uterus for testing or treatment. The counselor will also review the risk factors involved. If the patient opts to have an amniocentesis, the counselor answers questions and presents the necessary consent form to sign ahead of time.

Amniotic fluid surrounds and protects a baby during pregnancy. It contains fetal cells and various chemicals produced by the baby. A sample of amniotic fluid is tested for Down Syndrome (Trisomy 21) and spina bifida.

Amniocentesis can provide valuable information about the baby's health. Even so, it is an invasive diagnostic procedure that requires serious reflection before opting for it. Some risk factors include a higher risk of miscarriage, cramping and vaginal bleeding, and possible leaking of amniotic fluid. The genetic counselor reviews all contingencies about what is involved with and at stake when having the test. It is also important for patients to be prepared for the results. What if the baby has a genetic defect? Some patients don't want to know and others do. It is a very difficult decision to make and one that is very personal.

Genetic amniocentesis is typically offered when test results suggest a Down Syndrome pregnancy because an Alpha-fetoprotein blood result came back positive. Alpha-fetoprotein is a protein produced by the unborn baby and any abnormal results could result in a child with spinal bifida or Down Syndrome. The genetic counselor and physician as to the necessity of the amnio will review each case, but in the end the decision to have genetic amniocentesis is up to the patient.

Level II Ultrasound

After meeting with the genetic counselor the patient undergoes a comprehensive ultrasound, known as a Level II ultrasound, performed by the perinatologist. The perinatologist is the physician who cares for the fetus and high risks pregnancies.[193] The ultrasound is usually done around 11 to 16 weeks of gestation, when the fetus is developed enough to see all body parts well.

The perinatalogist will perform the Level II ultrasound and will look at the baby from head to toe, including the four chambers of the heart, the face, lips, and internal organs. Updated ultrasound equipment allows the physician to see everything. Some clinics use ultrasound units that are so advanced the baby can be seen in a 3D image, which really brings the unborn baby to life. The ultrasound determines if the baby is developing normally and is healthy. It is also possible to find out the sex of the baby if the patient wishes.

The physician will perform an amniocentesis and collects some amniotic fluid less than an ounce at this time. Amniotic fluid is the fluid that surrounds the baby and contains cells and Alpha fetoprotein, which will be sent to the lab and tested for any genetic risks that may have been indicated. A long fine needle is inserted through the abdominal wall to the amniotic sac, which is done by ultrasound guidance. Sometimes the woman's abdomen is injected with a local anesthetic. Once the needle is in the sac a syringe is attached and will withdraw amniotic fluid, which will be sent to the lab for testing. The color of the fluid is similar to urine and the amount removed will depend on what testing is performed. If the Level II ultrasound reveals complications with the pregnancy, the perinatologist will watch you closely throughout your pregnancy and monitor you with ultrasounds and future consults to discuss the risk for future pregnancies.

First Trimester Screen

There is another test in the MFM program, which is new and optional called First Trimester Screen, which is performed a little earlier than Level II between 11 to 13.9 weeks of gestation. This test is a separate ultrasound from the Level II. It is a noninvasive evaluation that combines maternal blood test with and ultrasound evaluation of the fetus. This test identifies chromosome abnormalities, including Trisomy 21 (Down Syndrome) and Trisomy 18 (Edward's Syndrome). The genetic physician will take a measurement of the fetus's neck called (nuchal fold) during the ultrasound. Fetuses that have an extra chromosome may have extra fluid at the base of the neck, which would make the neck larger. The neck is transparent at this time and the ultrasound can measure the amount of fluid. The timing of the test (age of the fetus) is very important, as the transparency becomes less as the fetus grows.

The blood test results combined with the measurement of the nuchal translucency and the gestational age of the fetus will give a risk factor of possibly genetic abnormalities. This test does not measure neural tube defects. A neural tube defect (NTD) is a common birth defect, which has an opening in the spinal cord or brain that occurs very early in the developmental stage of the baby and can be detected through an Alpha feto protein blood test.

It is important to note that the First Trimester Screen is a screening test and not a diagnostic test. This means the test does not determine if the baby has Down Syndrome.

Instead, the screening gives the probability that a baby may have Down Syndrome (Trisomy 21) or Trisomy 18. This probability is based on three factors: age, ultrasound results, and blood work. The First trimester screen can either alert the patient and her physician that there may be an increased risk factor for one of the chromosome disorders. On the other hand, it may show a low risk for these conditions. I want women to know of the risks factors of getting pregnant at a later age, but there are tests, which can give a risk factor, and, if the risk factor is high, further testing that can help diagnosis the condition.

The advantage of the First Trimester screen is that it is performed very early in the pregnancy and a low-risk result offers the patient great reassurance of a healthy pregnancy. This reassurance is so important when they are newly pregnant and are in a high-risk group, getting that "OK" is so important. A lot of women will stop further testing at this point.

Patients with high-risk results are counseled immediately regarding further testing. This might include Chorionic Villus Sampling (CVS) (that is, sampling the placental tissue) and amniocentesis, which renders a more definitive diagnosis. Chorionic Villus is placental tissue and taking a sample of this tissue can detect chromosomal abnormalities. This procedure can be performed at 10 to 12 weeks where as an amniocentesis is usually performed at 15 to 20 weeks gestation. The sample can be collected using a thin flexible catheter and can be placed vaginally through the cervix to the placenta or it can be collected with a long thin needle through the abdomen to the placenta using ultrasound guidance. The genetic counselor will review any risks factors of CVS testing.

Regardless of test result, anyone in the MFM program can be assured that she and her baby are being well cared for and watched closely.

MaterniT21 Plus: DNA-Based Down Syndrome test [194]

There is new testing for Advanced Maternal Age (AMA) patients for Down Syndrome and other chromosomal abnormalities and it is called MaterniT21 Plus test. MaterniT21 Plus is a noninvasive prenatal test for detecting fetal chromosomal abnormalities with a high degree of accuracy. MaterniT21 is a new DNA-based screening test that has a 99 percent detection rate for Down Syndrome with a very low false positive rate. The test requires a sample of blood from the mother and can be performed as early as 10 weeks gestation. The test reports out simple positive or negative results and are completed within seven days.

Let's have a quick genetic lesson

Chromosomes are structures in our bodies that contain genes. These chromosomes and genes instruct our body on how it grows and develops. You inherit genes from your father and mother. Most people have 23 pairs of chromosomes and the first 22 pairs are called autosomes and they are the same in both the male and female. The 23rd pair of chromosome is the sex chromosome and this distinguishes the male (XY) from female (XX).

If you look at results from a Karyotype it lists all 22 pairs of chromosomes and the order would start with number one and go through to 22. If you physician orders a chromosome analysis, which is a blood test, the lab is doing a Karyotype.

Some people are born with an extra copy of a chromosome or a missing chromosome. If there is an extra copy of a chromosome, which would make three copies in total (remember the chromosome is already a pair) then this is called Trisomy. This extra can cause genetic problems in the child.

MaterniT21 tests for the following Trisomies:
- Trisomy 21, known as Down Syndrome, has an extra copy on the 21st chromosome. Babies with Down Syndrome have delays in intelligence and development.
- Trisomy 18 known as Edwards's Syndrome has an extra copy on the 18th chromosome. Babies born with Edward's Syndrome have multiple birth defects and many don't survive after first few months of life.
- Trisomy 13 known as Patau Syndrome has an extra copy on the 13th chromosome. Babies born with Patau Syndrome have multiple birth defects and many don't survive after first few months of life.
- MaterniT21 can test for other genetic abnormalities, which can be discussed with your RE.

I spoke to an infertility office about this new test and found out that they have been testing all patients with

AMA and patients with known hereditary issues in their family. The patient has their consult with the genetic counselor that will discuss this test. They are testing at 10 weeks gestation and they also recommend doing an ultrasound to measure the nuchal translucency. An amniocentesis is recommended for patients that have positive results on their MaterniT21 Plus. The good news is that they have seen a drop in the number of amnioncenteses being performed since the availability of the first trimester screen and the MaterniT21 Plus tests.[195]

It is important to keep in mind no test is perfect! While results of this test are highly accurate, false negatives and false positives may occur in rare circumstances. The benefits and limitations for this test should be discussed with your RE.

Chapter 22
Donor Egg Program

If the patient has undergone several IVF procedures that have not resulted in pregnancy; and as age creeps up on her; the time has come when she may have to consider a donor egg program. Some centers have an age limit after which they discontinue IVFs[196] because statistics indicate the success rate is very low. Further, insurance companies will not pay for any further cycles unless the patient is using donor eggs.[197] Even in those instances where an older women proceeds, it is important to be aware that any patient who is, say, 43 years of age and uses donor eggs, is still considered to be at an advanced age and thus possesses increased risk factors during the pregnancy.[198]

The donor-egg program is similar to using a sperm bank (discussed in the next chapter) in the manner of choosing a donor and checking the donor's characteristics such as eye and hair color, age, weight and height, race, education, heritage and religion.[199] The donor egg program involves a strict screening process. Before being approved, the donor goes through an initial written screening: answering questions for pre-qualifications and then a face-to-face screening. They meet with a social worker and are tested for all blood tests including all genetic testing.

In the case of the donor-egg program, the couple chooses a donor for the eggs and they would use the husband's sperm to fertilize those eggs. The recipient being the wife would take the hormone medications to prepare her uterus in preparation for the IVF transfer. She would carry the embryo, unless she has complicating issues, such as scar tissue in uterus (severe endometriosis). In this case she would explore the possibility of surrogate who donates her eggs and carries the child. (In contrast, a gestational carrier only carries the child using the egg and sperm of the couple.) Fifteen percent of the IVF procedures using donor eggs are successful.

A donor-egg program is much more expensive then ordering sperm from a sperm bank because more is involved, including harvesting the eggs from the donor and preparing the recipient for transfer. One program I looked at breaks the fees into three primary components:

1. The fee paid to the donor for her inconvenience and time as well as the expense associated with her pre-screening;
2. The cost of the donor's IVF cycle and associated medication to retrieve her eggs;
3. The cost of the recipient's cycle to prepare her for the embryo transfers into her uterus.

A traditional fresh egg donor cycle can cost between $25,000 and $38,000 (a frozen egg cycle is approximately half the cost). In most cases insurance does not cover donor-egg procedures. So patients need to be aware that this option will be out-of-pocket.[200]

I include here an example of what this process involves to give you an idea of what to expect.[201]

About our Donors[202]

While they are reimbursed for their time and effort, most women's decision to become a donor is born of a desire to help another woman and her partner achieve their dream of parenthood. The majority of egg donor cycles performed at Shady Grove Fertility are anonymous. Our anonymous donors come to us through various sources, mostly through word-of-mouth referrals from our current and past donors. Every potential donor undergoes an intensive medical and psychological screening process before she is accepted into our program.

Donor Candidates

Any woman between the ages of 21 and 31, who is healthy and has a healthy family history, may be initially considered for egg donation. All egg donor candidates must complete a medical history and genetic question-naire that is reviewed by our staff. View the donor screening process below:

Donor Screening Process

Prior to completing the physical process of donating

311

eggs, potential donors undergo both medical and psychological screening.

Donor Qualifications
- Ages 21 to 31
- Good general health
- Normal weight range, a BMI of 18 to 28
- Nonsmoker
- High school graduate or proof of GED
- Resident [in Shady Grove's program] of MD, VA, DC, DE, WV, or PA.

Infectious disease blood work, including:
- HIV 1 & 2 Antibody Screen
- HIV NAT (Nucleic acid-based tests)
- Hepatitis B Surface Antigen
- Hepatitis B Core (total antibody)
- Hepatitis C Virus Antibody
- Hepatitis C Virus NAT (Nucleic acid-based tests))
- Treponema Pallidum (Syphilis – RPR – Rapid Plasma Reagin)
- Chlamydia trachomatis
- Neisseria gonorrhea

Genetic testing, including:
- Beta Thalassemia
- Bloom Syndrome
- Canavan Disease
- Cystic Fibrosis
- Familial Dysautonomia

- Fanconi Anemia Type C
- Gaucher Disease
- Tay Sachs/Hexosamindase A deficiency
- Mucolipidosis IV
- Niemann-Pick Disease Type A
- Sickle Cell Disease
- Spinal Muscular Atrophy
- Fragile X

The donors also undergo drug screening, ovarian function testing and psychological tests (in written and face-to-face sessions).

Donor Recruitment

Shady Grove Fertility staff personally recruits, screens, and matches nearly all of the egg donors in our anonymous donor program. Hands-on management of the egg donor recruitment is mutually beneficial to the donor and patient. The process allows us to:

1. Manage egg donor compensation - a cost paid for by the recipient.
2. Use local donors to eliminate out-of-pocket travel and related expenses.
3. Eliminate miscommunication caused by 3rd party coordination.
4. Offer donors and recipients confidence and peace of mind

The Donor Database

We are continually recruiting potential donors and

matching qualified donors with recipients. We have a large number of egg donors to select; including donors of various ethnicities.

Choosing Your Donor Option

- *Anonymous Donor:* Most women opt to undergo the egg donation process as anonymous donors. Their identity remains anonymous through out the whole donor process. The majority of women who donate their eggs anonymously are "recruited" donors.

- *Shared Anonymous Donor:* These are Anonymous Donors who have previously donated their eggs. They produced a high number of good quality eggs. The previous recipient had a successful cycle and or has embryos cryopreserved. Because of their previous successful cycle, we will choose to "share" this donor between two anonymous recipients. This option not only gives each recipient an equal chance of success in achieving pregnancy, it also means sharing the financial responsibility with the other recipient couple.

- *Known Donor:* Some couples will elect to use a relative such as a sister, cousin, friend, or others close to a recipient to assist them with this process. In addition, some recipients who are looking for a specific requirement that is not commonly found will sometimes opt to "self recruit" an egg donor by searching out prospective donors on their own.

- *Split Egg Donor:* These are women who also need

an assisted reproductive cycle (IVF) themselves and who are willing to "split" their eggs with you. (You get half, they get half.) Often these women do not have Insurance coverage for IVF or the financial means to pay for the IVF procedure. They are patients of the practice, and are referred to the program by one of our physicians. These women are offered participation in this program because the physicians feel they will produce a substantial number of good quality eggs thus giving both you and the donor an equal chance of success in achieving a pregnancy.[203]

This is a great example of a reputable and thorough donor-egg program wherein the donor is thoroughly tested. For the recipient couple, any and all of these steps require time and reflection to think through. I mentioned earlier in the book whenever another party becomes involved, whether through egg or sperm donation, it is important for all parties to seek help with a fertility counselor or psychologist. There is a lot to think about and they may be things you haven't thought about.

Chapter 23
Sperm-Banking, Freezing Sperm & the Non-donor Bank

Your RE may suggest that your male partner store some specimens in a sperm bank. (The industry vernacular ascribes this the verb form, "sperm-banking.") Your infertility clinic may offer the service, which is called a non-donor sperm bank, in which the male partner freezes his own specimens for his own use with his partner. (If your clinic does not offer this service then your nurse or RE will suggest the closest sperm bank in your area.)

Why would your RE suggest that you sperm-bank?

- Some men have careers in which they travel a lot and cannot be available when their wives are ready for an IUI or IVF procedure. (We had a patient who was an airline pilot and his schedule was work one week, home the next.) This takes the stress off of the couple worrying if the male is away when the procedure takes place. There is enough stress and to know there is sperm frozen is like an insurance policy in case the male is away.
- Some men experience performance anxiety when

expected to produce a specimen at a particular time. Banking some specimens settles the mind of the patient, being consoled that, when trying to collect a specimen and finds he can't, the option remains to use the frozen specimens.

- For those men who have with poor quality sperm, low count and low motility, freezing samples ensure the best possible outcomes during an IVF procedure if he produced fresh sperm that showed low quality or no motility. In that case the lab would ask for the frozen sample.

- Some men have certain types of cancer when they are young and may not have a partner at the time or family. The radiation and chemotherapy treatment kills the sperm. So by sperm banking at this time could give the young male patient a way of saving his fertility for a later date when he meets someone, they would come back to the sperm bank for his specimens.

For men who are reading this book please keep in mind: If for some reason you are diagnosed with cancer and may not yet have children, consider sperm-banking. The oncologist is focusing upon treating your cancer aggressively and may overlook the importance of preserving healthy sperm prior to treatment, since some cancer regimens affect fertility.

Procedure for sperm banking in a Non-Donor bank

For reasons explained above the couple may want to sperm-bank specimens. This involves calling the sperm-bank lab to make an appointment, at which time the lab explains all details of the procedure. The patients will call their insurance company to determine if it covers this procedure. There are many different charges associated with banking and the insurance company may pay for some, depending on the reasons for resorting to this. For example, if the patient is banking for infertility reasons only (not associated physical problems) he may be considered a short-term patient and bank for only one year. If he has cancer and is banking for that reason, he may be considered a long-term patient and the specimens can be stored up to 10 years.[204]

On the day of the appointment the patient brings a photo ID and any other identification required by the lab and then sits down to complete consent forms with the technician. In some cases the female partner is present to complete some of the consent forms as well.

The consents are typically legal documents that address being tested for STDs and what happens if any of these tests register positive. For example, if a test registers positive for Hepatitis B, these results go to the specialist so the female partner must then also be tested, since Hepatitis B can be passed on through intercourse. The sperm can still be used it just has to be stored in quarantine most likely at a commercial sperm bank.

Further, there is no guarantee that the freezing will result in a pregnancy, which will be addressed in the forms that will be filled out. There is a section in which the male partner is asked what would become of the frozen samples if something happened to the male partner, such as passing away or if male partner loses mental capacities.

He will have the choice of disposing of the specimens or leaving the specimen to the executor of his estate. In most situations the specimens are left to the female partner. Again if you don't have a partner because you are a young man that is sperm banking because of having cancer and you don't have a partner at the time of banking, you can leave the specimen to someone, such as a parent. Even so, this parent can only give it to someone you are sexually intimate with. For example, a 16-year-old patient has testicular cancer and will be receiving radiation. He wants to preserve his fertility through banking his sperm before the radiation treatment since the radiation will kill the sperm. At the time of banking the patient does not have a partner? Even so, he could leave his sperm to a parent in the case that he passes away. The parent can only assign the sperm only to a partner with whom their son could have been intimate with before he passed. Most patients in this situation will dispose of the specimens.

Once the consent forms are completed, the male partner produces a specimen and, depending on where the procedure is being done, the male has his blood drawn to test for STDs.

When the lab freezes the specimen, they measure your ejaculate, the total volume of the specimen produced along with a sperm count. Depending on the count they will add equal volumes of freezing media to the sample. The media protects the sperm during the freeze. Let's say that you produced 3 milliliters (ml) of semen from the first ejaculate. The medical technologist would then add 3 ml of freezing media to the sample, totaling 6 ml of fluid for freezing. The tech divides the 6 ml into one-milliliter vials for freezing. Thus, a single ejaculate renders six vials. An IUI procedure would use one vial; an IVF procedure may use two vials. So a single ejaculate could be saved for a few procedures.

The lab performs a post thaw test, which analyzes a small portion of the larger sample that is to be frozen. They will aliquot a small sample and freeze it. The following day they will thaw the vial and read it under the scope and they will count the motile sperm and non-motile sperm. The motility will drop about 25 to 30 percent from the original count before the freeze. This is normal, and if the motility drops significantly the lab may ask for another specimen, to be frozen.

If the patient has cancer, the clinic may try to bank as many ejaculates as possible before the treatment. Certain cancers affect the sperm count. If the patient has a low count as a result of cancer, there is no need to worry. If the sample numbers are low the ICSI (Intracytoplasmic sperm injection) procedure could be performed. This is where one sperm is injected directly into the egg. Some cancer patients may only have one to two vials frozen because of very low sperm counts. So to conserve the specimen for other procedures in the future the IVF labs can "shave a little off" the top of one of the vials, instead of thawing the complete vial. This small effort may render sperm so that the rest of the vial can stay frozen. Once a vial is thawed, it can't be re-frozen.

Once the specimens are frozen and all is said and done, the patient may have one-to-four ejaculates preserved, which equates six to 24 vials. The samples are stored in liquid nitrogen until needed. If the patient happens to re-locate the specimens can be shipped to another sperm bank or lab. The specimens have to stay frozen and you would see any infertility specialist at the new clinic.

Sperm bank typically charges an annual storage fee. At the time of this writing, the cost to freeze one ejaculate could be around $1,000.00 and the annual storage could be around $600.00.

Sperm banking is a service that helps patients keep stress levels down for both partners. It consoles the couple to know that, no matter what happens—travel or performance anxiety—they have a specimen to use. It's amazing to look under the scope and see the sperm come back after being frozen for years. I read a study[205] that was performed comparing fresh to frozen sperm for IVF procedures and there was no difference found in the pregnancy rate or number of live births.

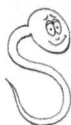

panky says:

"If you think your hands are too rough for collecting a specimen use a little hand cream to soften your hands for a few days before collection, since you can't use any cream that day."

Chapter 24
Freezing Eggs

As noted, lifestyles have changed for women. They are seeking careers and may be waiting before starting a family. The last chapter highlighted that sperm have been frozen for many years. Sperm has been frozen for over 50 years and embryos have been frozen over 30 years. The technique for freezing was a slow process wherein the tissues were exposed to cryoprotectants that removed the water from the cells and protecting the cells during freezing and thawing processes. Then the cells would be stored in liquid nitrogen and then thawed. This slow freezing process has been shown to have a good survival rate. This has been possible because the sperm is a small cell compared to an egg. The process is good for embryos and sperm, whereas eggs seem to be more sensitive to this type of freezing. The egg contains more water, which makes it harder to freeze on its own.

Until recently, egg freezing was an experimental procedure with limited success in only a few select programs around the world. However, the use of a specific type of freezing called vitrification, has led to a dramatic improvement in oocytes survival, fertilization rates, and pregnancy rates. Most importantly, these successes are being reported by many different centers worldwide.[206]

The principle is simple. This new method of cryo-preservation allows ultra-rapid freezing. The eggs in very small droplets of vitrification solution in special straws, and plunge them directly in liquid nitrogen. This means the egg is cooled from 37 C to -196 C in a few seconds, so that the water does not get a chance to crystallize! Vitrification uses a very high concentration of antifreeze solution Dimethyl Sulfoxide (DMSO) and (ethylene glycol) allowing instant super-cooling into solid with no ice crystal formation at all.[207]

Of course, it is not quite as simple as it might sound. Such high concentrations of antifreeze could be toxic to cells. This is why technical skill, experience and expertise are critically important.

Using the vitrification technique for freezing, we can reliably preserve eggs as well as embryos so that the pregnancy rate is as good as with fresh eggs.

This breakthrough allows infertility clinics to offer the following additional services to their patients:

- Formation of donor "egg banks" to facilitate and lessen the cost of oocyte donation. We can ship these frozen oocyte anywhere in the world. However, it is critically important that the receiving IVF lab have enough expertise in vitrification, to be able to thaw these properly.
- Allow for cancer patients to preserve their fertility before their chemotherapy or radiation treatment makes them infertile or go into menopause early.

- Provision of egg cryostorage for women who wish to pursue their career and want to postpone child-bearing.[208]

There is controversy over the last service, which freezes eggs for women who want to stop their biological clock. Freezing eggs is a very new technique and anything that is new sometimes met with skepticism and a wait-and-see approach. The American Society for Reproductive Medicine issued a statement recently: "The ASRM points out a problem that women freezing eggs to put off motherhood still have an age issue. Most of the women who are freezing their eggs are in their mid to late 30s and their eggs have already started to age thus starting to be less fertile. They also feel elective egg freezing an experimental procedure has insufficient data on usage and outcomes to assure patients it's a worthwhile undertaking."[209]

The two most common reasons to consider egg freezing include, first, stopping the "biological clock." For the first time in history a woman can prevent her age from affecting her fertility since the eggs are removed from the ovaries, then frozen, and these eggs do not age. Another reason to freeze eggs is to preserve fertility in woman about to undergo chemotherapy and/or radiation.

I read an interesting article[210] about successful professional women in New York who were successful in their careers and who hadn't found Mr. Right yet. They confronted the dilemma: Do I freeze my eggs at 30 years old in order to come back to them when I am 40 and have the baby then?

Egg freezing is a luxury that costs anywhere between $10,000 to $15,000. The women who are having this procedure are very successful women who have felt stuck between the mixed messages that "the 40s are the new 30s" and that the biological clock is ticking and it is important to have children before the age of 35 years.

It is important to keep in mind, however, that even if a woman freezes her eggs at a younger age, there are no guarantees she will get pregnant. Often it is the case that, as women get older they become more set in their ways and wait longer to find a life's companion – perhaps possessing an idealized notion of what Mr. Right might look like. Add that a career, perhaps schooling, and before you know it, the biological clock is really ticking away.

Here is one scenario worth thinking about: a woman had cancer and did a couple of IVF cycles with her boyfriend at the time. As a result they kept a number of frozen embryos. She survived the cancer, however her boyfriend was married to someone else. Now she confronts the dilemma, does she use these embryos? Her doctor told her that, even after her cancer treatment, she still had her fertility and her eggs were good. She was in no rush and wanted to find Mr. Right. So she made the decision to freeze her eggs with the hope that, after she finds the right relationship she will start a family.

Freezing your eggs is an ever-changing scenario and not every woman can do this. As always, it is a matter of the patient doing what is right for her and what she feels good about. She must be content with her decision.

Chapter 25
Fertility During Cancer Treatments

There are many types of cancers diagnosis that may affect young people before they even have a chance of thinking of children and their fertility. For patients who find themselves in the position, remember that as the oncologist discusses the form of treatment for your particular type of cancer, they tend to be more involved in the treatment than they are about preserving the patient's fertility, male or female.

Most treatments for cancer – chemotherapy, radiation (or both) and/or surgery – can leave patients with infertility problems in the aftermath of the treatment. It is extremely difficult to comprehend the diagnosis of cancer, let alone the thoughts about your fertility. However, patients must be aware of the consequences of cancer treatments and consider options that won't adversely affect future fertility. During cancer treatment the patient must consider the effects: blood work, computerized axial tomography CAT scans and positron emission tomography PET scans. Preserving fertility should also be in this category.

How to Preserve Fertility During Cancer Treatments
The following section comes directly from medical

oncologist, Dr. Gauri Bhide: [211]

"This is an important question to address during treatment planning, as all potential chemotherapy can cause infertility in both men and women. Most of the malignancies that affect people in their young childbearing ages are potentially curable and the possible effect on future childbearing needs to be discussed.

Men have a long-tested (and used) option of storing frozen sperm. Sperm banks and the technology for banking are commonly available. Sperm count and motility will be tested before storage to make sure that there is enough viable sperm. In prepubescent males the possibility of storing testicular tissue for future re-implants is being explored, but is not mainstream.

Women in a stable relationship have the option of freezing embryos, similar to the process for IVF. However, they now also have the option of freezing oocytes, or eggs, in the absence of a sperm donor. The freezing of ovarian tissue for re-implantation is being used in select centers. This is experimental in prepubescent girls and all re-implantation carries some risk of re-implanting cancer cells.

Harvesting of eggs used to take at least a month and there was reluctance to delay the initiation of curative chemotherapy. This can be now achieved with a seven-day cycle as per reproductive endocrinologists.

If fertility is restored naturally, with normal sperm

count and function, and normal menstrual cycles with ovulation, there does not appear to be any greater risk to such offspring as a result of treatment, so it is not necessary to use the stored sperm and eggs. However, resumption of menstrual cycles does not mean resumption of ovulation.

When to discuss fertility preservation?

There is so much happening with a new cancer diagnosis that the preservation of fertility takes a back seat. However, with high cure rates and long life expectancy this needs to be offered as part of treatment planning. The timeliness of the process can be facilitated if there exist lines of referral and communication with sperm banks and reproductive endocrinologists.

I have a lovely anecdote of a 27-year-old woman who was going through fertility issues before her diagnosis of Hodgkin's lymphoma. At that point, they were not interested in additional procedures for fertility given her difficulty in conceiving to begin with. We completed her curative chemotherapy, she resumed normal menstrual cycles, and a few years later, had given birth to two naturally conceived children! I also have many patients who have happily adopted children to complete their families. And I have many others who have chosen not to pursue either."

Chapter 26
Same Sex Couples & Surrogacy ART

In the past 30 years, the gay rights movement has increasingly encouraged gay men and women not only to be open about their homosexuality and about their relationships, but also to be open about choosing to have children. News is wide and rampant everywhere with the ongoing evolution in laws regarding same sex marriage. This inevitably introduces the element of raising a family for these now legally married couples.

Some same-sex couples have families from their previously heterosexual relationships. Others have families through adoption. More recently, however, many gay couples are expressing interest in becoming parents together and establishing a "traditional family" in the context of their same sex union.

This, however, brings about some difficulties. A few states prohibit same-sex couples from adopting, particularly in Utah and Mississippi. Further, some religious groups refuse providing adoption services to them.

Even so, some of these couples still want families, despite the obstacles. They are seeking parenthood through Assisted Reproductive Technology (ART). Lesbian couples in the past have been routinely treated in fertility clinics for the obvious reason that such procedures are easier, since females have the eggs and can carry the child. Now gay men, however, are also seeking help for becoming parents through various fertility centers. In the case of gay men, it means seeking out an egg donor as well as a surrogate.

Lesbian Couple or Single Woman

The lesbian couple determine ahead of time which partner will carry the child. This could be based upon age, any prior infertility treatments. Or the decision could be based upon what simply works best for the couple socially or professionally. Which partner could more easily attain maternity leave? Which has the better insurance? It is also possible that the original plan may change based on if test results came out poorly. In this case the other partner may opt to be the one getting pregnant. Once they've determined who will carry the pregnancy, they would undergo an initial consult with the RE. At that point, the RE may want the couple to see an infertility counselor for any further questions they may have regarding their specific situation.

The female patient would then go through the same pre-testing regimen that Mary had completed (See Chapter 9): the Clomid challenge test, blood work, hysteroscopy, and Hysterosalingogram (HSG).

In turn, the nurses give the couple information on various Commercial Sperm banks where they can explore possible donor sperm. (The commercial sperm banks have web sites where the interested parties can view all characteristics of their sperm donor.) The same holds true if a single woman, with no partner, wants to have a child. (Many single women with careers are beginning to recognize that their biological clock is ticking away.) She too would meet with the RE and have the same preliminary testing performed. Then, she too would look into Commercial Sperm banks for donor sperm.

How a Commercial Sperm Bank works

Sperm banks are called cryobanks. These cryobanks enable single woman and lesbian couples to acquire donor sperm. They also help heterosexual couples, if for example, the male partner has a genetic condition that makes him infertile. (Sperm banks also enable men to bank their sperm for their own use for those who are getting radiation or chemotherapy, which kills the sperm.)

Donors

There are many sperm banks in the United States and these banks are usually located near universities where many intelligent (so-called "smart sperm") and viral men live. (A high percentage of donors are college students, though others come from all walks of life.)

Men donate to a sperm bank for a variety of reasons. Whatever the motivation, all donors go through the same screening process, which takes approximately a year. To become a sperm donor thorough semen and blood tests are performed, as well as a physical exam. The donor will also complete a very extensive medical form which he will list all of his family history. Potential donors have to pass strict criteria for semen parameters and blood testing before being accepted, and not every man is able to become a donor. The sperm bank tests all candidates for Sexually Transmitted Diseases (STDs) such as HIV, Hepatitis, HTLV I and II (Mediterranean disease) and more. Donors are also being tested for genetic disease such as Cystic Fibrosis, Fragile X and Tay- Sachs.

Some sperm banks may also have requirements for height, age (18 to 38 years), and level of education. Sperm banks can make their own criteria for what they want for donors.

The FDA has stepped into the realm of sperm banking and they impose very strict regulations when it comes to donor sperm because they want to make sure that all specimens are safe from any sexually transmitted diseases to protect the recipients. The donor will also need to supply many semen specimens to make sure his specimen is normal and has a strong count, motility and a normal morphology. The specimens need to be consistently the same with the semen results. (People are purchasing these specimens, so the sperm bank wants a good specimen. The bank keeps track of pregnancy results, so a recipient could inquire when they pick a donor to find out how many women were able to be pregnant from that particular donor.) Once a donor passes the testing requirements and the blood and urine work is negative, his specimens will be quarantined for six months. Then, at six months, the donor will undergo a second set of testing for STDs. (There is a six-month window for some

STDs wherein a patient can be negative the first time tested but positive six months later.)[212]

I suggest choosing a sperm bank that provides genetic counselors. All women seeking a donor should make an appointment with one of them. The counselor will go over family history to see any genetic issues the recipient may have and answer any questions on selecting a donor. Further, some recipients may ask for additional genetic testing on the donor because of their own family medical history.

When searching for donors, patients you can choose from hair color, eye color, race, blood type, medical history and family history. Sperm banks may offer packages for a fee that will include baby pictures, audio clips where the donor is interviewed and you will be able to hear the donor and this will help you get to know more about him. When a donor is qualified he will get a donor number – for example, D 334. This number will stay with this particular donor forever. The process for the donor is easy. He goes to the sperm bank and collects a specimen by masturbating into a sterile specimen cup and he is paid anywhere from $ 40.00 to $100.00 for each sample. A donor can collect many specimens over a year or less. Even so, there is a limit to the number of children a donor can produce and each country has laws on according to the number of children. The reason for this is to limit sperm donations in the risk of accidental inbreeding between offspring. In some countries limits are voluntary and while others have a law.[213]

When a patient searches for a donor, some sperm

banks list medical information and STD results. There is one test called Cytomegalovirus (CMV), which may show positive for the donor. CMV is a very common virus, which infects approximately 70 percent of people up to the age of 45 years and up to 90 percent to the age of 80 years. In most cases the initial infection show no symptoms and with others they feel like they have flu like symptoms. After the initial infection the virus stays dormant in the body. If the immune system becomes weakened in the future there is a chance the virus will reactivate. If a patient is interested in a donor who has tested positive for CMV and wonders if this donor is safe, the answer is yes. The screening test that is done for CMV can determine if it is a past infection or an active infection. Only donors with past infections can be kept and any donor with a current infection will be destroyed. If you have any questions please speak to your RE if you are interested in a donor that shows a positive result for CMV.

Once the recipient has selected a donor, you are ready to order your samples. Just like everything in infertility terminology can be confusing so it is important to understand how to order your samples. The sperm bank processes the donor specimens in two ways because one process is good for IUIs and the other is good for IVF cycles. For example, if your RE were starting you with IUIs, you would order a washed sample or intrauterine insemination (IUI ready). If you are doing an IVF cycle you would order an unwashed specimen or intracervical insemination (ICI ready), Let me explain more about each process:

Washed specimen v. Unwashed specimen

Back in Chapter 17 I talked about the IUI procedure and how the semen specimen was washed before the insemination. Remember for a semen specimen to be placed in the uterus, the sample must be washed. In sperm banking the same process occurs. The complete specimen from the day of collection is washed, and then a cryoprotectant is added to the sample, it is separated into little sterile vials and then the vials get frozen in liquid nitrogen. This specimen is called a washed specimen or an IUI ready specimen for a Donor Insemination (DI), which is one way to process a sample.

If a patient is doing IUIs at a clinic this is the sample to order. The cost for the sample is higher but it is considered "ready to go." What do I mean by that? The day the patient is having the insemination the sample will come out of liquid nitrogen about 20 to 30 minutes beforehand. The sample is thawed and the lab will perform a sperm count motility test and you'll have your procedure called Donor Insemination (DI). As mentioned earlier some women's OB-GYN will start with some infertility treatment and some may do IUIs for their patients. In this case the patient would either bring the frozen specimen in a shipper to the office or have the specimen delivered on the day of the IUI/DI and this would be a washed specimen.

The other process, the complete sample has cryoprotectant added directly to the sample and then separated in little vials and then frozen. It does not go through the washing procedure and this process is called unwashed or ICI ready. Intracervical insemination (ICI) was done years ago before IUI. The difference is, the semen specimen that was not washed was placed in front of the cervix as opposed to going through cervix to the uterus. ICIs were performed before the new technique of washing sperm came about. Sperm banks use the terminology of ICI as another term, which means the specimen was not washed. When you are doing IVF cycle the embryology lab would prefer ICI or unwashed specimens. The IVF lab has their own procedure on preparing the sperm for IVF, so they like the specimen unwashed.

By now you are asking, can it get anymore confusing? Yes!

The sperm bank has both types of specimens on hand when a patient calls to place an order. Sometimes, depending upon the donor, there may be only ICI specimens with no IUI left. That's Okay! If a patient orders an ICI (unwashed) and she is doing IUIs at the clinic, the lab can wash the ICI vial before the procedure. When a patient is doing an IUI with an unwashed specimen it takes longer to process than an IUI-ready specimen, so it is important to keep this in mind. Patients communicate to the nursing staff what type of specimen has been purchased.

It is incredible to think that sperm can be frozen for years and once thawed are moving around like they were collected that day. The cryoprotectant protects the sperm during the cold storage of liquid nitrogen for those years.

Things to keep in mind:

Once a sample is frozen and the vial is removed from liquid nitrogen (thawing process) the sample has to be used within a short period of time (hours). The sample can't be taken out and refrozen, the sperm won't survive.

Sperm counts are performed for total sperm numbers and motility before and after the freeze. (A small sample is frozen separately and counted the next day to get a count of how the sperm took the freeze)

Every time a procedure is done to a sample including washing or freezing the percent (%) motility of the sperm will drop. They all can't live through it, but using donor sperm – these samples should be very potent and that is why the donors are tested quite a few times before being qualified to become a donor.

Before proceeding, the patient will want to ask the sperm bank how many vials does a particular donor have, considering as well, the possibility of future children having the same donor. If a patient purchases extra vials, she will need to pay yearly storage fees at that particular bank.

Some banks allow the donor to remain anonymous or to stay anonymous until the child reaches 18 years of age. This is called an open-identity donation. Those donors who choose to have an open identity have the choice about when and how to communicate with their offspring. Each sperm bank has differing policies and it is up to the donor to decide what he wants to do. Families and recipients do like the option to identify the donor so their child can meet their biological father at some point in their life. The donor has no legal bearing on the children. Another point to keep in mind is that other clients in the same general vicinity could use the same donor.

The donor you choose can go to anyone.

I saw a television program called *Who's your Daddy?* – a television documentary highlighting the story of a sperm donor who donated specimens while he was in law school, and had fathered 72 children. He had registered on a Donor Sibling Registry that matches children conceived by sperm donors with their biological father and half-siblings. The T.V. documentary showed the donor meeting two of his children with their mother. At the time of the airing of the television program he was planning his wedding and mentioned to his fiancée that the number was up to 70. His fiancée was not happy about the situation. It is something to think about! She said, " What if they all come knocking?" The donor was glad to have helped so many families.

In the USA, there are no regulations governing who may engage in sperm donation. The American Society of Reproductive Medicine provides recommendations and guidelines. The ASRM guidelines limits a donor to have 25 live births per population of 850,000, although this is not tracked or enforced by law, and it has been estimated that 40 percent of births are reported.[214]

Below is a list of commonly asked questions while choosing a sperm donor:

- Should the donor possess physical characteristics similar to my own or my partners?
- Do I want to use an opened-identity donor?
- Can I have more than one child from this donor?
- What is the donor's medical and family history?

- What type of person is the donor? Hobbies, education, interests etc.?
- How many pregnancies have occurred with this donor?
- How many vials does this donor have?

During the course of infertility treatment, after the patient has selected the donor, the sperm is shipped to the center for the time when the specimen is needed for either the IUI or IVF procedures. Since most centers do not have storage to keep patients frozen vials, the patient is responsible to have the vial or vials shipped as close as possible to the date of the procedure. Typically, one vial is used for the IUI while the IVF lab may want two vials shipped for the IVF procedure. The sperm bank ships the sperm in a canister containing liquid nitrogen to keep the specimen frozen lasting up to five-to-seven days. (The patient should check with the sperm bank to be confirming this.) Once the specimens are thawed they need to be used and they can't be refrozen.

It is your responsibility to call the sperm bank and set up the shipping arrangements and you will pay for the charges at that time. The patient needs to choose the shipping schedule carefully so as not to fall on a weekend and the patient should not wait until the day before the procedure to ship the samples.

I have encountered situations in our lab when patients shipped sperm in a particularly stormy winter. One weekend a woman showed up for an IUI and we didn't have any sperm. It came to light that the patient ordered only one sample, during her last cycle, and didn't realize she had to call for another sample each month and that it is not automatic. It can get very confusing.

Directed Donor

Some choose to have a directed donor. This arrangement serves those women who want sperm from someone they know, but with whom they are not intimate, like a good friend. Even so, women need to understand the potential problems that can occur in this case, if she chooses to go this route without using the proper channels. There are potential health risks -- sperm through IUI can transmit infectious disease such as HIV, Hepatitis and other STDs even when intercourse is not involved. Further, there are also laws concerning parental rights that both parties need to understand.

A directed donor would still have to go to a commercial sperm bank to be tested for STDs and his sperm would be quarantined for six months. FDA regulations have changed and the quarantine period can be less than 6 months but the donor may have to do additional testing. Then he would be re-tested for STDs and as long as everything was negative his samples could be shipped to your Infertility clinic. The quality of the sperm will be evaluated also to make certain that you have the best chance of becoming pregnant.

In addition to the possibility of spreading an infectious disease and the uncertain quality of the sample, the legal aspects remain quite important. When a friend gives his sperm to get a woman pregnant, he does not want parental rights. When a man donates his sperm through a sperm bank and the recipient receives the sperm through a physician, he relinquishes all parental rights, including financial responsibility for the child. Since laws don't specify receiving sperm from a friend through IUIs, the potential exists for paternity problems in the future. If sperm donation is not done by means of the proper channels, a mother can ask the donor for child support. Each state differs on this situation.

There was a recent case in which a lesbian couple used sperm from a directed donor, choosing not to go through a sperm bank or a licensed physician for the IUI procedure. The recipient successfully gave birth to a child. The couple later filed for state assistance, and the state required the name of the donor in order to collect child support for the child (who was now three years of age). The state contended that the agreement between the couple and donor was not valid because state requires a licensed physician to perform artificial insemination. This is still in court. The result may well be that the directed donor will have to pay child support. This example underscores the complex nature of sperm donation because of the many parties involved. It is very important that the patient considers these contingencies and works hard to make sure everything is done properly and legally to avoid these kinds of complication.

What is Surrogacy?

The word "surrogate" means substitute or replacement. Within infertility treatment, a surrogate mother is one who lends her uterus to another couple so that they can have a baby.[215] Surrogacy is when a third party woman enters into a legal agreement to carry and give birth a couple's baby, There are two types of surrogacy:

Traditional Surrogacy: Traditional surrogacy is where a woman donates her eggs and carries the child. She is the genetic mother of this child. This woman would do an IVF cycle where she would take the FSH injections to stimulate her ovaries to produce eggs. The eggs would be retrieved and placed in a petri dish with the intended husband's sperm or donor sperm. The embryo(s) would then be transferred back into the woman and she would carry the embryo(s) to delivery.

Gestational Surrogacy: Gestational surrogacy is where a woman only carries the embryo(s) and delivers the baby. There is no genetic relationship. This woman would take medications to prepare her uterus for transfer of the embryo(s) that were created by the husband and wife and carry the baby through the pregnancy and delivery the baby.

Who would need surrogacy treatment?

Some women may have a medical condition that makes it impossible for her to carry a child. Or, she may have been born without a uterus. Others may have had their uterus removed because of excessive bleeding during a caesarean section.[216] There are also woman that can get pregnant but have recurrent miscarriages. There are some women who go through a number of failed IVF cycles, which leaves scar tissue in their uterus. This is another situation that would make it difficult for an embryo to implant and making surrogacy an option.

In the case of gay male couples, they are increasingly expressing the desire to become parents together and establishing a "traditional family structure" in their relationship. Many have become fathers through adoption or perhaps have children who were conceived when they were in a heterosexual relationship. Many of these couples are looking at becoming fathers through ART— that is, IVF—and using an egg donor and a gestational surrogate or a traditional surrogate that would donate her eggs and carry the baby.

Do your homework

Any patient who is considering surrogacy must always explore all the legal aspects first in order to avoid legal contingencies that may arise later. States look at several factors when establishing parental rights and these include genetic ties, delivery of the baby and the intended parents. Any of these aspects are considered factors in determining parental rights. Traditional surrogates possess two of these factors. It sometimes arise that when the baby is delivered the surrogate mother finds herself incapable of giving up that baby. A person may have a good friend who says she is willing to donate the eggs or to be the surrogate; she will say that she is fine about it and will have nothing to do with the baby. Even so, once that baby is born, these women often experience an unexpected life-changing bond with the baby and, for that person; all previous assurances evaporate, ruining the friendship. (Often it is stipulated that if someone wants to become a surrogate, the candidate must first have a child or children of her own.) It is important also to understand that infertility centers connect patients to egg donors, sperm donors and surrogates, but they do not give legal advice. For this reason it is very important to get lawyers involved and look at and understand the state laws first.

Despite the emotional complicating elements to surrogacy, there are some heart-warming stories. I spoke to a patient one day who explained to me how she was a surrogate for her sister. I asked her would she tell her story for the book and she was very happy to do so:

When I got married in 2007, I never envisioned what was going to happen in the years following the wonderful day. We were blessed with a beautiful baby boy in the spring of 2010 and we couldn't have been happier. My older sister had struggled with infertility for nine years and then had a stroke in 2009. The doctors informed her that her heart wouldn't be able to sustain a pregnancy. When my son was three months old, my sister and I were getting manicures, she casually mentioned looking into surrogacy. I'll never forget sitting there letting my nails dry and I offered to be her surrogate. She was shocked and told me that is was a huge decision. I went home that afternoon, and my husband said, "of course, I want to help them too." People have asked me several times why I offered without thinking it through. I looked at it as if I was offering my sister an organ. If she needed a kidney, I would never hesitate. This time, she needed a uterus.

My husband was supportive and we went ahead with the treatments to get the uterus ready for my sister's embryos. My sister used her eggs and her husband's sperm and the embryos were transferred to my uterus. We were all surprised and filled with joy, when we found out that I was carrying twin girls. I will never regret the decision to become a surrogate because I am able to see the joy that my nieces bring to my sister and her husband. I feel more in love with my husband because he was my rock. I am looking forward to the day when we tell my son and nieces about how they entered the world. I think it's a true testament of the love of a family.

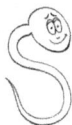

Conclusion
When Do You Stop Infertility Treatment?

I had a male patient who, when dropping off a semen analysis, indicated he wanted to talk to someone. I happened to be there and he felt comfortable trusting me with his thoughts (it must have been my big blue eyes). He started to explain to me that he and his wife have a beautiful healthy child who was conceived naturally. They had been trying for a second child through natural conception, which didn't happen. When he and I spoke they were in their second year of infertility treatment and still not pregnant. He spoke of his desperation in trying to talk with his wife about the possibility of stopping at one?

It was clear to me that she wanted more children and in this way, I explained to him how important it is to keep communicating and to try and understand that, in her mind, one more treatment may be necessary before she can accept the circumstances. It can happen with a lot of couples that one wants to keep trying while the other feels there has been enough stress and that it is time let go of the process. Each person involved in this complicated and emotional process has his or her own time.

Couples need to try and understand each other's feelings and give each other the space and safety they need. The process should never devolve to the place where the couple is arguing and have stopped supporting one another.

If a patient or couple finds themselves faced with a decision about when to end fertility treatment, but are not sure how to go about finalizing it, there are steps to take. It is helpful to begin the process with a pre-determined time frame in mind. Some patients take a vacation from treatments and come back feeling rejuvenated. Some realize that the time has come to look into a different option or that it is time to stop. It often happens that couples decide to begin the adoption process and then all of a sudden they get pregnant. It happens.

Infertility can feel like an endless series of tests and treatments and at some point patients will have to let go and grieve; come to closure and allow resolution. It is a great help to talk to others who have faced this decision and have moved on. It helps to know you are not alone. Professional counseling also can be very helpful. Finally it is important to recognize that infertility will always remains a part of a patient's story. The decision to stop treatment may bring closure and resolution, but it may not remove altogether the pain of infertility. Even so, once the decision is made people often find that the disappointment disappears.[217]

I asked our nurse Sandy what happens to unsuccessful patients? She said, "Unsuccessful patients sometimes just disappeared and never talk to us about stopping treatment. The ones who do talk to us would get information about adoption, if they were interested. Sometimes they get other opinions at other programs to see if they had anything different to offer them. The organization Resolve[218] has programs on when to stop treatment that can help couples make that decision."

Adoption

There are many different choices to be made for adoption. One of the first decisions is whether to adopt from the United States (a domestic adoption), or from another country (an intercountry adoption). Other considerations include deciding on the importance of the child's medical and genetic history and how much contact you may want to have with the child's birth family. The U.S. Department of Health and Human Services has a very helpful website that includes a fact sheet to educate families about adoptions.[219]

Joining a Medical Registry?

The National Institute of Health (NIH) has funded the creation of a nationwide research pool of current and former infertility patients. The Infertility Family Research Registry (IFFR), helps centralize information on infertility and gives families a way to learn about research studies and provides researchers a way to find research participants. The IFFR adds medical knowledge that helps other infertility patients; assists in studies of infertility and mental health, newborn and child development; and improves treatment of infertility in the U.S. All information is kept confidential and patients who participate are helping others.[220]

Acknowledgements

I've have been working in the infertility field for over 12 years and not only seeing a need for the book, but the patients I've met over the years are the nicest and sincere group that truly want to have a family and that is why I wanted to write *Sperm Tales*. I have had many mentors who have helped me with learning and working in infertility but I have a few very special people to thank in writing *Sperm Tales*.

My loving husband Kevin helped me so much in 1997. He helped start the lab: specimens are not easy to obtain when you need to test out your equipment. Kevin was also a great help with ideas and helped me solve problem areas within the book.

I was very fortunate to work with one of the best Reproductive Endocrinologists in the field, Dr. Mitchell Scott Rein. I remember our first meeting and discussing what his expectations were for the lab. I never met a nicer person and boss to work with. He loved his job and showed this in a very caring way with his patients. Our head nurse, Sandy Vance, came from Boston and has a lot of experience in the infertility field, she has worked in California years ago where infertility first started. Sandy has such compassion for her patients and work hard to have a wonderful nursing team.

My administrator, Julie Kautz Mills, has to be the best person to work with. Julie helped me through the ups and downs. I've always been a lover of biology and science and to be working in such an advanced and growing field, I feel very fortunate. Julie was the one who named Spanky!

I have to say, in the course of writing this book I have met many wonderful, caring physicians and specialists in their field around the world. *Sperm Tales* was started in 2009 and I'm finishing it six years later. The research was the major part and talking to reproductive specialists, urologists and other specialists has been incredible. The minute they found out that I was writing a book to help patients in an Infertility program, they jumped at the chance to help me.

I wanted to thank each one of them:

One of my first specialists I contacted and has been such a tremendous help was Dr. Aniruddha Malpani, MD, from Bombay, India. Others I want to acknowledge: Dr Jay S. Nemiro; Connie Shapiro, Ph.D from Psychology Today; Dr Laurence A. Jacobs, M.D.; Dr Samuel Marcus; Dr Janice L. Andreyko; Dr. Stephen Wells; Dr. Charles W. Monteith; Dr Mark Perole; Michael A. Werner, M.D.; Stanton C. Honig M.D.; Dr Stanley Ducharme Ph.D; Scott Roseff, M.D.; Donald Evenson, Ph.D; Dr. Sergio Oehninger; Dr Gauri Bhide; Laurence A. Jacobs M.D., Dr. Stephen Hudson , Abraham Kryger, M.D.; Dr. Stephen Lazarou; Zhenzhen Zhang, Acupuncturist; Paula J Wilson, Yoga Instructor; Bill Simms from WEBMD; Shady Grove

Fertility Center; Shared Journey fertility website.

I need to give special thanks to my editor Wendy Murray, who I was fortunate to learn about through a dear friend. Wendy is a seasoned award-winning journalist, author and editor who has published many books. I have always felt *Sperm Tales* was in good hands as she and I worked closely together.

The drawings were reproduced by Justin Coburn.

I hope that *Sperm Tales* will help everyone and you'll be seeing more of Spanky.

Acronyms

2WW: Two Week Waiting
AFP: Alpha Fetoprotein
AMA: Advanced Maternal Age
AMH: Anti-Mullerian Hormone
ART: Assisted Reproductive Technologies
ASRM: American Society for Reproductive Medicine
BBT: Basal Body Temperature
BMI: Body Mass Index
CAH: Congenital Adrenal Hyperplasia
CAP: College of American Pathologists
CAVD: Congenital Absence of Vas deferens
CCT: Clomid Challenge Test
CDC: Centers for Disease Control
CISA: Clinical Immunization Society Assessment
CM: Cervical Mucus
CMV: Cytomegalovirus
CT, CAT: Computed Tomography
CVS: Chorionic Villus Sampling
D & C: Dilation and Curettage
DFI: DNA Fragmentation Index
DHEA: Dehydroepiandrosterone
DI: Donor Insemination
DMSO: Dimethyl Sulfoxide
DNA: Deoxyribonucleic Acid

DOR: Diminished Ovarian Reserve

DVD: Digital Video Disc

E2: Estradiol

ED: Erectile Dysfunction

ER: Emergency Room

eSET: Elective Single Embryo Transfer

ESHRE: European Society of Human Reproduction and Embryology

FDA: Food and Drug Administration

FET: Frozen Embryo Transfer

FSH: Follicle Stimulating Hormone

GIFT: Gamete IntrafallopianTransfer

GnRH: Gonadotropin-releasing Hormone

GTD: Gestational Trophoblastic Disease

HA: Hyaluronic Acid

HCG, hCG: Human Chorionic Gonadotropin

HIV: Human Immunodeficiency

HMG: Human Menopausal Gonadotropin

HPV: (Genital) Human Papilloma Virus

HSG: Hysterosalpingogram

HTLV: Human T-cell lymphotropic virus

IAAC: Infertility Awareness Association of Canada

ICI: Intracervical Insemination

ICSI: Intracytoplasmic Sperm Injection

ID: Identification

IFFR: Infertility Family Research Registry

IM: Intramuscular (injection)

IUD :Intrauterine Device

IUI: Intrauterine Insemination

IV: Intravenous

IVF: InVitro Fertilization

LH: Luteinizing Hormone

LPD: Luteal Phase Deficit

MESA: Microsurgical Epididymal Sperm Aspiration

MFM: Maternal Fetal Medicine

ML: Milliliter

MTHFR:Methylenetetrahydrofolate Reductase

MRI: Magnetic Resonance Imaging

NAT: Nucleic Acid Test

NGU: Nongonoccal Urethritis

NT: Nuchal Translucency

NTD: Neural Tube Defect

OBGYN: Obstetrician/Gynecologist

OHSS: Ovarian Hyperstimulation Syndrome

OPK: Ovulation Predictor Kits

PCOS: Polycystic Ovary Syndrome

PED: Performance Enhancing Drugs

PESA: Percutaneous Epididymal Sperm Aspiration

PET: Positron Emission Tomography

PGD: Preimplantation Genetic Diagnosis

PID: Pelvic Inflammatory Disease

PMS: Premenstrual Syndrome

RE: Reproductive Endocrinologist

ROS: Reactive Oxidative Species

RPR: Rapid Plasma Reagin

SART: Society for Assisted Reproductive Technologies

SC: Subcutaneous (injection)

SCSA: Sperm Chromatin Structure Assay

SHBG: Sex Hormone Binding Globulin

SRRS: Social Readjustment Rating Scale

STD: Sexually Transmitted Disease

TESE: Testicular Sperm Extraction

TNF: Tumor Necrosis Factor

TSH: Thyroid Stimulating Hormone

VAERS: Vaccine Adverse Event Reporting Systems

VSD: Vaccine Safety Datalink

VZV : Varicella Zoster Virus

WHO: World Health Organization

ZIFT: Zygote Intrafallopian Transfer

ZP: Zona Pellucida

Glossary of Terms

Acrosome - the anterior portion of the sperm head, which contains enzymes that break down the outside shell of the egg during fertilization.

Adhesions - scar tissue that may be located in the abdominal cavity, fallopian tubes, or inside the uterus that can interfere with the transport of the egg and implantation of the embryo in the uterus.

Agglutination - the term used when sperm are stuck together either by head-to-head, tail-to-head or tail-to-tail.

Advanced Maternal Age (AMA) - the term used for women getting pregnant over the age of 35. The risks for problems with the baby and the pregnancy increase as a woman's age increases.

Amenorrhea - the lack of a menstrual period for six months or more.

Amniocentesis - a prenatal test, which removes a small amount of amniotic fluid from the sac around the baby in the uterus and is used to test for any genetic abnormalities.

Androgens - any of a group of hormones that primarily influence the growth and development of the male reproductive system.

Andrology - the medical speciality related to functions and diseases of men's health, particularly infertility, urology and sexual dysfunction.

Aneuploidy - is a variation in chromosome number that involves individual chromosomes. There may be fewer or more chromosomes ie, Down Syndrome has 3 copies instead of 2 copies on chromosome 21.

Anomaly - an abnormality in any part of the body.

Anovulation - the failure to ovulate; a common cause of infertility in women.

Antibody - a protective protein produced in the body that fights or otherwise interacts with a foreign substance in the body.

Anti-Mullerian Hormone (AMH) - fertility testing that gives an estimate of the remaining egg supply or ovarian reserve; blood is tested on any day of the cycle.

Antiphospholipid Syndrome - an autoimmune state caused by Antiphospholipid antibodies that can cause blood clots in the body as well as pregnancy complications as miscarriage, stillbirths or implantation results.

Antisperm Antibodies - proteins (antibodies) that fight a man's sperm in blood, vaginal fluids, or semen; can cause the sperm to stick together.

Antral follicles - ovarian follicles at a very early stage of growth; there are ways to test the number of follicles, which will give a women's ovarian reserve (also called resting follicles or "good" follicles).

Asherman's Syndrome - a condition characterized by adhesions or scarring inside the uterus or the cervix; often the front and back of the uterine walls stick together, occurring when there is trauma to the uterine tissue triggering the wound healing process that causes the damaged areas to fuse together.

Assisted Hatching - a micromanipulation procedure in which an opening is made into the hard outer surface of the early embryo with the use of chemicals, mechanical techniques, or lasers to improve implantation after the embryo is transferred into the uterus.

Assisted Reproductive Technology (ART) - is the technology used to achieve pregnancy in procedures like fertility medications, artificial insemination and in vitro fertilization.

Azoospermia - when there is a complete absence of sperm in the ejaculate.

Basal Body Temperature (BBT) - the temperature at which your body is fully at rest and during ovulation there is a slight increase in this temperature; used to help determine ovulation.

Beta HCG Test (hCG) - see HCG.

Bicornate Uterus - a congenital malformation of the uterus in which it appears to have two horns.

Blastocyst - a stage of embryonic development that occurs about five days after fertilization.

Blastocyst Transfer - also known as Day-5 transfer, when the blastocyst stage embryos are placed in the uterus.

Body Mass Index (BMI) - a simple index of weight and height that is commonly used to classify underweight, overweight and obesity in adults.

Cervical Mucus (CM) - is a fluid that is secreted by the cervix, the production of which is stimulated by estrogen. Throughout the menstrual cycle the amount and quality of cervical mucus changes and by observing these changes can help you predict the most fertile days of your cycle.

Cervix - the narrow neck like canal forming the lower end of the uterus.

Chlamydia - a sexually transmitted disease that can impair infertility.

Chorionic Villus Sampling (CVS) - prenatal testing for genetic disorders (such as Down Syndrome), which uses a sample of placental tissue; can be performed between 10 to 12 weeks of gestation.

Chromosomes - rod-shaped bodies in a cell's nucleus that carry the genes that convey hereditary characteristics; made up of DNA.

Clomiphene (Clomid) - a non-steroidal fertility medicine that causes the pituitary gland to release hormones needed to stimulate ovulation (the release of an egg from the ovary); Clomid is used to cause ovulation in women who did not ovulate regularly.

Clomid Challenge Test (CCT) - a test to check ovarian reserve consisting of a Day 3 blood FSH followed by oral medication Clomid on Days 5-9, then being retested for blood on Day 10.

Coitus Interruptus - sexual practice in which the penis is withdrawn prior to ejaculation to prevent the deposit of sperm into the vagina.

Conception - the process of becoming pregnant by the fertilization of an egg by sperm and implantation, which results in miracle of a baby.

Congenital - conditions present from birth, either hereditary or environmental.

Congenital Absence of Vas Deferens (CAVD) - a condition in men where the tubes (Vas deferens) that carry the sperm out are missing or fail to develop properly before birth. There can be one tube missing (unilateral) or two tubes missing (bilateral). Vas deferens carry the sperm from the testicle to the penis.

Congenital Adrenal Hyperplasia (CAH) - a group of genetic disorders of the adrenal gland; the condition means bodies are lacking an enzyme needed by the adrenal glands to produce the hormones cortisol and aldosterone.

Corpus Luteum - a yellow-colored cyst that forms from the ovarian follicle after it releases an egg; the cyst produces estrogen and progesterone to prepare and support the uterine lining for implantation.

Cryobank - also known as Sperm Bank, collects and stores donor sperm from women in need of donor sperm to become pregnant.

Cryopreservation - a procedure used to preserve (by freezing) and store embryos or gametes (sperm, oocytes).

Cryptorchidism - a condition of undescended testicles.

Dehydroepiandrosterone (DHEA) - a steroidal hormone produced by the adrenal glands that is able to turn into other steroidal hormones (estrogen and testosterone); women who experience diminished ovarian reserve (DOR) as a result of a slow or inactive adrenal gland and lack naturally occurring DHEA need to be closely monitored when undergoing DHEA replacement therapy.

Dilatation and Curettage (D & C) - dilatation of the cervix to allow scraping of the uterine lining with an instrument (curette); removes tissue from the uterus after a miscarriage or removing pieces of placenta after birth.

Diminished Ovarian Reserve (DOR) - a decrease in the quantity or quality of oocytes (eggs), leading to infertility.

Directed Donor - an individual who stores sperm for a designated recipient who is not sexually intimate with the recipient.

DNA Fragmentation Index (DFI) - measures the integrity of the DNA in the sperm nucleus, and is associated with a positive or negative pregnancy outcome.

Donor Insemination (DI) - an Assisted Reproduction Technique using donor-frozen sperm deposited directly into the uterus, bypassing the cervix, and allowing the sperm to enter the fallopian tubes.

Donor Sperm - semen specimens donated to a sperm bank and used in an IUI or IVF procedure.

Ectopic Pregnancy - a pregnancy in which the fertilized egg implants anywhere but in the uterine cavity (usually in the fallopian tube, the ovary or the abdominal cavity).

Egg (Oocyte) Donation (Donor Egg) - the surgical removal of an egg from one woman after ovarian hyper-stimulation for transfer into another women using partner's sperm with IVF procedure.

Egg Retrieval - a procedure used to collect eggs from women's follicles for use in IVF.

Ejaculation - the male orgasm during which approximately two to five milliliters of semen (seminal fluid and sperm) are ejaculated from the penis.

Elective Single Embryo Transfer (eSET) – the primary goal of eSET is to reduce multiple pregnancy rates that are associated with IVF. Transferring more than one embryo could result in multiple pregnancies.

Embryo - term used to describe the early stages of fetal growth from conception to the eighth week of pregnancy.

Embryo Grading - the embryologist will look at the petri dishes under the microscope and grade each embryo according to quality of their appearance, cell number and cell regularity, assigning the embryo a grade according to its quality.

Embryologist - a scientist who studies the formation, early growth and development of human embryos.

Embryo Transfer - the introduction of an embryo into a woman's uterus after IVF.

Endometriosis - the presence of endometrial tissue (the normal uterine lining) in abnormal locations such as the tubes, ovaries and peritoneal cavity, often causing painful menstruation and infertility.

Endometrium - the mucous membrane lining the uterus.

Epididymis - a coiled, tubular organ attached to and lying on the testicle where the sperm are stored and matured before ejaculation.

Erectile Dysfunction (ED) - the inability to keep or get an erection firm enough to have sexual intercourse.

Estradiol (E2) - a type of estrogen, the major sex hormone in women, released by the developing follicles in the ovaries; injectable medications stimulate the ovaries to produce more follicles, which increase estrogen in the blood. Blood is drawn to measures estradiol levels to determine the progressive growth of the follicle during ovarian stimulation.

Estrogen - a major female hormone, produced mainly by the ovaries from the onset of puberty until menopause, also responsible for the development of secondary sexual characteristics in women.

Fallopian Tubes - a pair of narrow tubes that carry the ovum (egg) from the ovary to the body of the uterus.

Fertility Clinic - a program of fertility specialists offering a range of fertility services, usually including ART.

Fertilization - penetration of the egg by the sperm cell.

Fertilization results - when the embryologist looks at the petri dishes that contain the eggs and sperm a day or two after the egg retrieval and counts how many eggs fertilized.

Fetus - a term used for the developing baby after the 8th week after conception until the moment of birth.

Fibroid - a benign tumor of fibrous tissue that may occur in the uterine wall; may be totally without symptoms or may cause abnormal menstrual patterns or infertility.

First Trimester Screen - a prenatal test that offers early information about a baby's risk of certain chromosomal conditions including Down syndrome (Trisomy 21); the test combines a sample of the maternal blood along with an ultrasound evaluation of the fetus neck (nuchal translucency).

Flare Protocol - a protocol for patients who have responded poorly during ovarian stimulation and did not produce a good number of eggs; involves Lupron being started earlier in the cycle, which produces an initial "flare-up" response of FSH and LH release from the woman's pituitary gland (a kind of "jump start" for the ovaries to produce more follicles).

Follicle - fluid-filled sac in the ovary that has nurtured the ripening egg from which the egg is released.

Follicle Stimulating Hormone (FSH) - a hormone produced in the anterior pituitary that stimulates the ovary to ripen a follicle for ovulation.

Frozen Embryo Transfer (FET) - transfer of an embryo, which has been frozen, from a previous fresh IVF cycle and then thawed and transferred into the uterus.

Gamete Intra-Fallopian Transfer (GIFT) - an ART procedure in which the sperm and eggs are transferred by laparoscopy into the fallopian tubes where fertilization takes place.

Gene - a segment of DNA that is passed down from parents to children. Genes are organized and packaged in units called "chromosomes." Humans have 23 pairs of chromosomes, 46 in total. One set of chromosomes comes from the mother and the other set comes from the father. These genes makes up who we are today as individuals.

Genetic Abnormality - disorders arising from an anomaly in the chromosomal structure, which may or may not be hereditary.

Genetic Counselling - advice and information provided, usually by a team of experts on the detection and risk of recurrence of genetic disorders.

Genetics - is the study of genes and heredity.

Gestation - the period of fetal development in the uterus from conception to birth, usually considered to be 40 weeks in humans.

Gestational Carrier (Surrogacy) - see Surrogacy.

Gonadotropin Releasing Hormone (GnRH) Agonists - drugs that inhibit premature ovulation.

Gynecologist (OB-GYN) - a physician who specializes in the health of women and the female reproductive system.

Hormone - a chemical substance produced in the body that controls and regulates the activity of certain cells or organs.

Human Chorionic Gonadotropin (HCG, hCG) - a hormone secreted by the placenta during pregnancy and it is measured in a blood test used to detect very early pregnancies to evaluate the development of the embryo. It is also a medication used to trigger ovulation.

Human Menopausal Gonadotropins (HMG) - a medication given to women who don't ovulate on their own and have pituitary deficiencies with hormone production; contains FSH and LH and will stimulate ovaries to produce follicles.

Hyaluronic Acid (HA) - a substance that is naturally present in the human body found in highest concentrations in fluids in the eyes and joints. HA is present in the cell membrane around the egg, which helps attract the sperm to the egg for fertilization.

Hyperprolactinemia - excessive prolactin levels which can occur in both females and males causing infertility.

Hypothalamus - a part of the brain that regulates hormones, located next to the pituitary gland at the base of the brain.

Hysterosalpingogram (HSG) - an X-ray of the pelvic organs that injects a radio-opaque dye through the cervix into the uterus and fallopian tubes, to check for malformations of the uterus or blocked fallopian tubes in suspected infertility.

Hysteroscopy - a surgical procedure to check for abnormalities within the uterus. Placing a small, thin telescope-like instrument called a hysteroscope through the cervical canal to inspect the inside of the uterus; used both to diagnose and treat problems.

Implantation - the process of attachment of the embryo to the maternal uterine wall.

Infertility - the inability to conceive after a year of unprotected, well-timed intercourse, or the inability to carry a pregnancy to term.

Insulin Resistance - a physiological condition wherein the natural hormone, insulin, becomes less effective at lowering blood sugars; the resulting increase in blood glucose may raise levels outside the normal range and cause adverse health effects and can be seen in women with PCOS.

Intracervical Insemination (ICI) – similar to an IUI but the sperm are placed near but not inside the cervix. This is an ART technique which was common in the 1980s.

Intracytoplasmic Sperm Injection (ICSI) - an IVF procedure where a single sperm is injected through the egg to cause fertilization.

Intramuscular Injection - an injection given into a muscle.

Intrauterine Insemination (IUI) - an Assisted Reproduction Technique which deposits washed sperm directly into the uterus, bypassing the cervix, and allowing the sperm to enter the fallopian tubes (where fertilization normally occurs).

In Vitro Fertilization (IVF) - is an Assisted Reproductive technology that manually combines the egg and sperm together in glass petri dishes and then transfers the embryo(s) back into the uterus.

Karyotype - a genetic test that examines chromosomes in a sample of cells, which shows the number and visual appearance of the chromosomes and help identify any genetic abnormalities.

Klinefelter's Syndrome - a genetic condition in a male where there is an extra X chromosome, so he would have XXY; this may be evident in pea-sized hard testicles and enlarged breasts

Laparoscopy - a minimally invasive surgical procedure in which a telescope-like instrument called a laparoscope is inserted through a small incision in the abdominal wall to view the inner organs in order to diagnose and sometimes treat suspected reproductive problems.

Level II Ultrasound - an ultrasound, which is performed

between 11 and 16 weeks gestation. The physician gives an extensive scan of the baby from head to toe and focuses on specific organs like the heart, brain, kidneys and other organs.

LH Surge - a sudden large release of luteinizing hormone from the pituitary glad triggers the almost ripened egg to become fully mature and break through the follicle (24- 36 hours after the surge the ovulation occurs releasing the ripened egg into the fallopian tube).

Lupron - a medication that is given during the IVF protocol to prevent ovulation before the desired time in the egg retrieval.

Luteal Phase - the second half of the menstrual cycle that occurs between the release of an egg and the menstrual period.

Luteinizing Hormone (LH) - a pituitary hormone that stimulates the ovaries or testicles. In females an acute rise of LH triggers ovulation. This is the hormone that the ovulation predictor kits measure in your urine

Male Factor - a term used for any problems in the production of sperm, anatomy of male reproductive organs or problems with the male's immune system, which causes infertility in the male.

Maternal Fetal Medicine - an obstetrical program that focuses on complicated high-risk pregnancies.

MaterniT21 Plus - new testing for Advanced Maternal Age (AMA) patients for Down syndrome and other chromosomal abnormalities, done with a sampled of blood at 10 weeks gestation.

Menstrual Cycle - is the monthly cycle of natural changes that occurs in the uterus and ovary as an essential part of reproduction averaging 28 days.

Micromanipulation - the use of high magnification and special instrumentation on microscopes to manipulate sperm, eggs, and embryos during IVF.

Microsurgical Epididymal Sperm Aspiration (MESA) - is a delicate process by which sperm is aspirated using a microscope and taken from an area close to the tubal blockage.

Miscarriage - the spontaneous loss of a fetus before the 20th week of pregnancy. Another term for miscarriage is a spontaneous abortion.

Mock Embryo Transfer - a procedure to measure the angle and depth of the patient's cervix, uterus and the thickness of uterine lining before embryo transfer to ensure the actual embryo transfer proceeds smoothly, optimizing the embryo implantation; the procedure eliminates potential problems that may arise during the first IVF cycle.

Molar Pregnancy - is also called a Gestational Trophoblastic Disease (GTD) and a hydatidiform mole. A molar pregnancy occurs when a genetic error occurs during fertilization and causes an abnormal growth in the uterus.

Non-Donor Sperm - frozen sperm donated by intimate partner, which would be used for IUI of IVF procedure.

Neural Tube Defect (NTD) - a common birth defect, wherein an opening in the spinal cord or brain occurs very early in the developmental stage of the baby and can be detected through an Alpha feto protein blood test.

Nuchal Translucency (NT) - an ultrasound test that measures the nuchal fold thickness of the neck of the unborn baby; one of the components of the first trimester screen along with maternal blood can aid in the early detection of Down syndrome and other genetic abnormalities.

Oligospermia - the term for a low sperm count in the ejaculate.

Oocyte - the biological term for an egg cell.

Orchitis - swelling or inflammation of one or both of the testes caused by many types of bacteria or viruses, the most common of which is mumps.

Ovarian Cyst - a fluid-filled sac within or on the surface of the ovary.

Ovarian Hyperstimulation Syndrome (OHSS) - a complication occasionally seen in women who take certain fertility medications that stimulate egg production. Ovarian hyperstimulation can cause ovarian enlargement and discomfort and fluid can leak into the abdominal area.

Ovarian Reserve - refers to a women's current egg supply and is closely related to the reproductive potential. The greater number of remaining eggs, the better chances with conceiving. Conversely, low ovarian reserve diminishes the chances for conceiving, also known as diminished ovarian reserve (DOR).

Ovulation - the release of a mature egg from a follicle.

Ovulation Stimulation - drug treatment that stimulates the development and release of one or more mature eggs from the ovaries.

Ovulation Predictor Kits (OPK) - kits that measure the hormone LH that increases when ovulation occurs and a positive test indicates the most fertile time of the month.

Papanicolaou (PAP) Smear - a microscopic examination of cells scraped from the cervix to detect cancerous or pre-cancerous conditions of the cervix.

Pelvic Inflammatory Disease (PID) - a general term for infection of the female reproductive organs.

Percutaneous Epididymal Sperm Aspiration (PESA) - a process by which a needle is placed in the epididymis where sperm are stored and matured and epididymal tissue is removed for IVF-ICSI.

Perinatalogist - an obstetrical sub-specialist concerned with the care of the mother and fetus at higher-than-normal risk for complications.

Pituitary Gland - a small gland found at the bone of the brain that secretes many hormones, including FSH and LH.

Polycystic Ovary Syndrome (PCOS) - a common condition affecting five to ten percent of women. It occurs when there is an imbalance of hormones that regulate the menstruation cycle and cause a failure to ovulate. The imbalance also shows itself in the increase of the male hormones, called androgens (including testosterone).

Preimplantation Genetic Diagnosis (PGD) - a new advanced reproductive technology used in conjunction with IVF for diagnosis of genetic disease in the embryo(s) before transferring them back to the patient. It is being used widely in most IVF centers and has increased the success rates for an IVF pregnancy in couples that have had previous IVF failures.

Premature Ejaculation - uncontrolled ejaculation either before or shortly after sexual penetration.

Progesterone - an important ovarian hormone that is normally secreted after ovulation and during pregnancy; progesterone triggers thickening of the lining of the uterus so it can accept implantation of a fertilized egg.

Prolactin - is the pituitary hormone that stimulates the production of milk in breast-feeding women. It also circulates in low levels in the bloodstream of non-pregnant women. High levels of prolactin in non-pregnant women can cause anovulation.

Prostate Gland - the gland encircling the urethra in men that produces a third of the fluid in the ejaculate.

Reactive Oxidative Species (ROS) - are chemically reactive molecules that contain oxygen. ROS are formed by the metabolism of oxygen. Environmental stress can increase the ROS which will damage cell structure. Oxidative stress is a main contributor to sperm DNA fragmentation.

Reproductive Endocrinologist (RE) - an obstetrician-gynecologist who has completed additional training in reproductive endocrinology. Reproductive endocrinologists are qualified to manage imbalances in the complex hormonal reproductive system, including infertility and recurrent pregnancy loss.

Retrograde Ejaculation - a condition that causes the semen to be ejaculated into the bladder rather than out through the urethra because of the failure of the bladder sphincter to close during ejaculation.

Semen - fluid of the male reproductive tract containing sperm and a number of other substances such as water, simple sugars, alkaline chemicals, and prostaglandins.

Semen Analysis (SA) - a laboratory test used to assess the amount and quality of a man's sperm and semen.

Seminal Vesicles - sac-like pouches that attach to the vas deferens near the base of the bladder; seminal vesicles produce a sugar-rich fluid (fructose) that provides sperm with a source of energy to help them move.

Sexually Transmitted Diseases (STD) - infections passed from one person to another through sexual, oral, or anal intercourse; through sharing needles; mutual masturbation; or general contact with infected bodily fluids. Some examples of STDs are Hepatitis, HIV, Herpes, Chlamydia, Gonorrhea, Syphilis and Genital Human Papillomavirus (HPV).

Sperm - the microscopic cell that carries the male's genetic information.

Spermatogenesis - sperm production.

Sperm Bank - a facility that collects and stores human sperm from sperm donors for use by women who need sperm to become pregnant.

Sperm Count - the number of sperm in the ejaculate, also called sperm concentration and given as the number of millions of sperm per milliliters.

Sperm Morphology - the evaluation of the size and shape of sperm in a semen sample.

Sperm Motility - the ability of sperm to swim.

Sperm Wash - a lab procedure used to separate sperm cells from the seminal fluid, which is used for artificial insemination.

Sterility - a condition that results in the inability to reproduce.

Subcutaneous Injection - is an injection that is given just under the skin.

Surrogacy - the word "surrogate" means substitute or replace. Traditional surrogacy is when a woman donates her eggs and carries the child and is the genetic mother of this child; Gestational surrogacy is when a woman only carries the embryo(s) and delivers the baby, having no genetic relationship.

Testicles - also known as testes, testicles are the male sex glands located in the scrotum; testicles store and produce sperm and are the main source for the secretion of the male hormone testosterone.

Testicular Biopsy - a surgical procedure in which a small sample of testicular tissue is removed for microscopic examination to see if sperm are present and able to be retrieved. See TESE, PESE.

Testicular Injury or Torsion - sports injuries can cause injury to the testes or torsion. Testicular injuries can be very serious and cause bruising, internal bleeding to one or both of the testes. If the spermatic cord becomes twisted (torsion), this is considered a medical emergency. When testicular torsion occurs the blood flow is cut off to the teste and surrounding tissue and can cause the tissue to die.

Testicular Sperm Extraction (TESE) - a process in which a small portion of testicular tissue is extracted that contains viable sperm usable for the IVF - ICSI cycle.

Testosterone - the primary male hormone responsible for secondary sex characteristics and for supporting the sex drive; testosterone is necessary for sperm production.

Tubal Ligation - a procedure, which causes female sterility. The fallopian tubes are blocked to prevent the egg from meeting sperm; commonly known as "having the tubes tied".

Ultrasound - uses of high-frequency sound waves that are reflected off solid tissues to give an image of internal body structures. This device is used to detect and count follicle growth in many fertility treatments and to detect and monitor pregnancy.

Unwashed Specimen (ICI ready) - donor or non-donor sperm that has been frozen with cryoprotectant, but is not washed.

Urologist - a physician that specializes in the urinary tract for females and male and also specializes in the male reproductive tract.

Uterus - part of the female reproductive system that contains and nourishes a fetus prior to birth.

Varicocele - an enlargement of the veins with in the scrotum; the scrotum is the tissue sac that holds the testicles. Varicoceles can be a cause in low sperm production, quality that can cause infertility.

Vas deferens - a coiled duct that transports the sperm from the epididymis to the urethra.

Vitrification - a new freezing technique for eggs and embryos, which provides the benefits of cryopreservation without damage to the cells due to ice crystal formation.

Washed Specimen (IUI ready) - donor or non-donor sperm that has been through a sperm wash and then frozen.

Zona Pellucida (ZP) - a thick transparent membrane surrounding the outside of the egg and this structure helps the sperm penetrate the egg during fertilization. It is the same membrane that surrounds the embryo, which is thinned out during Assisted hatching to aid the embryo in implantation.

Zygote - an embryo in the early stages of development.

Zygote Intrafallopian Transfer (ZIFT) - a type of Assisted Reproductive Technology in which the female's eggs are mixed with the sperm of the male partner in a dish in the embryology lab. The fertilized eggs, called zygotes, are then transferred within 24 hours into the fallopian tubes.

Endnotes

1. Ref: CDC, Centers of Disease Control and Prevention, Assisted Reproductive Technology (ART), Section 5: ART Trends 2000-2009, Is the use of ART increasing? http://www.cdc.gov/art/ART2009/section5.htm

2. Claudia Kalb, "The Truth about Fertility," *Newsweek* August 13, 2001.

3. Kalb, Ibid.

4. In 2011 I was dining out on a few occasions I asked a group of young people this question. It's a small survey of 15 people, but I felt it was worth saying to show the thoughts of young people.

5. Some assert that for women who have been on the pill for an extended period of time, the age to start consultation drops to the upper 20s. A study in Italy was published in 2001, which says that fertility declines with women in the late 20s and not what we thought to be in the 30s. A male's fertility starts to drop in the late 30s. This is not to say couples can't get pregnant, but that it may take longer to get pregnant and they may have to seek help from an infertility program. And as you heard the saying, "Some of us don't always follow the book" meaning some may not have any problems getting pregnant.

6. "The Biological Clock," and originally aired on 4/7/2002.

7. I was married early in my twenties and quickly got divorced. It was one of those too-young marriages that shouldn't have happened. I found my current husband at 30 years old and we married when I was 33. I promptly went to the infertility specialist I

worked for and tried a few IUIs that did not succeed.I am lucky to have an understanding husband who was fine with not having children if that was the case. After another year of infertility treatments I did not get pregnant. Twenty years later I look at my life andI am happily married and have plenty of nieces and nephews to love.

8. Each clinic should also have statistics on their IUI success rate, which you should also request.

9. A cycle could be cancelled if the patient doesn't respond to the drug stimulation, meaning they didn't produce any follicles; the cycle can be cancelled if they over-respond the drug therapy (IUI cycle) and produce too many follicles. The RE doesn't want the patient to have too may children (a litter).

10. A study was published in Fertility and Sterility, a publication of the American Society of Reproductive Medicine, shows that women who participate in a mind/body program for stress reduction (discussed in the next chapter) while undergoing IVF treatment have a significant higher pregnancy rate than those who do not. (52 percent versus 20 percent)

11. *The New Harvard Guide to Women's Health,* Karne Carlson, MD; Stephanie Eisenhart, MD; Terra Ziporyn Ph.D. Social Adjustment Reading Scale, accessed , 10/17/12, p. 574. This is the resource where I mention the SSRS scale on level of stress.

12. Shady Grove Fertility Center, Rockville MD, Questions to ask Insurance companies for coverage. http://www.shadygrovefertility.com Ref; Janet L. Kaminski, Associate Legislative Attorney, INSURANCE COVERAGE FOR INFERTILITY TREATMENT, March 1, 2005; www.cga.ct.gov/2005/rpt/2005-R-0236.htm

13. Ref; Janet L. Kaminski, Associate Legislative Attorney, IN-SURANCE COVERAGE FOR INFERTILITY TREATMENT, March 1, 2005; www.cga.ct.gov/2005/rpt/2005-R-0236.htm; Massachusetts's law for covered treatments include artificial insemination (AI), In-Vitro Fertilization (IVF), Gamete Intra-Fallopian Transfer (GIFT), sperm, egg, or inseminated egg retrieval, Intra-Cytoplasmic Sperm Injection (ICSI) for male infertility, and Zygote Intra-Fallopian Transfer (ZIFT). The Massachusetts infertility insurance mandate also specifies that insurance companies cannot impose limitations, restrictions, or exclusions on coverage for fertility treatment drugs that are different from those imposed on other prescription drugs.

14. For complete information on insurance coverage go to the following site: http://www.resolve.org/family-building-options/insurance_coverage/state-coverage.html

15. The Family Act of 2011, S 965/H.R. 3522.

16. Connie Shapiro, Ph.D., "When You're Not Expecting: Infertility Counseling," *Psychology Today*, May 21, 2010; http://www.psychologytoday.com/blog/when-youre-not-expecting/201005/infertility-counseling-getting-started. Used with permission.

17. Constance Hoenk Shapiro, Wiley; 1 edition (February 8, 2010)

18. http://www.resolve.org

19. Ibid., Connie Shapiro

20. Gametes are reproductive cells that unite during reproduction. The male the gamete is the sperm and the female gamete

is the egg.

21. When I first heard the situation it sounded like the male was a "directed donor" A directed donor is a male that will give his sperm to a female because she may know him as a friend and want the sperm, but they are not sexually intimate. But this wasn't quite the case. The RE said that the three would have to see the clinic's therapist to discuss their situation and talk about the consequences of bringing up a child in their situation.

22. This is not to be confused with polysexuality, which is an attraction towards multiple genders.

23. As of July 2009, it was estimated that more than 500,000 polyamorous relationships existed in the United States. By law a polyamorous relations is no different than people who date or live together. (Wikipedia) http://en.wikipedia.org/wiki/polyamory.

24. Genital TB has a very high incidence in India and other countries: it is rarely encountered in the US. The lungs are the most common organs involved but TB is a systemic illness and any organ in the body can be affected. The disease is caused by a bacterium called Mycobacterium tuberculosis. These bacteria are spread by droplet infection that means it's in the air and spread by a cough or sneeze from an infected patient. The female genital organs are one of the common sites in women. It is a chronic disease and bacteria will remain for long time slowly destroying the organs. The disease may remain totally symptomless or may lead to pelvic pain, fever, menstrual disturbances or vaginal discharge. Infertility may be caused even by early or minimal disease.

25. Check first with your nurse to ascertain if any of these alter-

native therapies are available at your clinic of choice.

26. Paulus W, et al. Influence of acupuncture on the pregnancy rate in patients who undergo assisted reproduction therapy. Fertility and Sterility April 2002;77(4):721-4. "Pins and needles. Could acupuncture help promote pregnancy?" ABCNews. com, April 16, 2002. Dieterle S, Ying G, Hatzmann W, Neuer A: "Effect of acupuncture on the outcome of in vitro fertilization and intracytoplasmic sperm injection: a randomized, prospective, controlled clinical study," *Fertil Steril* 2006; 85(5): 13, 47-51. Westergaard LG, Mao Q, Krogslund M, Sandrini S, Lenz S, Grinsted J: "Acupuncture on the day of embryo transfer significantly improves the reproductive outcome in infertile women: a prospective, randomized trial," *Fertil Steril* 2006; 85(5): 13, 41-6. Smith C, Coyle M, Norman RJ: "Influence of acupuncture stimulation on pregnancy rates for women undergoing embryo transfer," *Fertil Steril* 2006; 85(5): 1352-8. Article written by :Zhenzhen Zhang, Lic. Acupuncturist http://www.acuherbalcare.com

27. Atzori, M. G. (2013). BSc, MS, DSHomMed, Women's Health Educator & Natural Fertility Expert.

28. Ibid., Atzori,

29. Wilson, Paula J. (2013). Registered Yoga Teacher, Amesbury, MA. website: www.harmonyyoga.info

30. Ibid., Wilson.

31. Ibid., Wilson.

32. Prounounced RAY-kee; reference: "Getting Pregnant and Natural Fertility: Reiki Therapy," http://www.gettingpregnant. co.uk/natural_fertility/reiki_therapy.html

33. Article from *ADVANCED* for Nurses, written by Pamela Giannatsis, November 24, 2003.

34. Injectables cost approximately $2,000 to $3,000 more than Clomid, including the price for bloods and ultrasounds. Medical insurance will pay this for some patients.

35. Dr Laurence A. Jacobs, M.D., Fertility Centers of Illinois, http://www.infertilitydoc.net/. OHSS will be discussed more in detail further along the book.

36. The bulk of this chapter is taken from ivf-infertility.com written by Dr Marcus Last Updated June 26, 2012 4:56 p.m. GMT.

37. The viral load is a measurement of the severity of the viral infection in your body. When you first have an infection of HIV, Hepatitis B or C the viral load is high. As the patient is treated, the viral load drops.

38. With the great success of IVF (test-tube baby) the chances are much higher for multiple births. This will be discussed further in the IVF section)

39. Mary also would need to set up an appointment for a Hysteroscopy and a Hysterosalpingogram (HSG), best done during the first week after her period. This would be set up after Mary makes the initial call to know when to set the appointment for the following week. The nurses will set up an HSG at the hospital and let Mary know when the test can be done.
40. Information in this section is derived from Kathleen Cahill Allison, American Medical Association, *Complete Guide to Women's Health*, (Random House, New York, 1996), "Menstruation," 204-209.

41. If you go to this site you will enter your previous menstrual cycles and it will give you your fertile time: http://www.webmd.com/baby/healthtool-ovulation-calculator.

42. Go to www.WEBMD.com and put in your menstrual dates to find out your fertile window. You will also want to use ovulation predictor kits to help detect when you are ovulating.

43. Some patients have trouble reading the OPK because of the color or intensity of color and can't decide if the test is positive or not. In this case, the nurses would have the patient come in everyday for a blood LH level to be drawn and the nurse would call you when your LH surged.

44. If you are aware of this discharge you may be able to take a sample of the mucus and stretch it between your fingers and note the color and consistency. The mucus appears thick sticky during non-fertile time and as your approach ovulation the mucus changes and becomes stretchy and pliable between your thumb and index finger.

45. Information in this paragraph comes from Dr. Aniruddha Malpani, MD, Malpani Infertility Clinic, Bombay, India, http://www.drmalpani.com/book/chapter16.html, accessed 10/14/2012.

46. This section is based upon Kathleen Cahill Allison, American Medical Association, Complete Guide to Women's Health,, (Random House, New York, 1996), Temperature Method 329-330.
47. Merck. Reviewed by Debbie Bridges, MD on August 21, 2009 © 2009 WebMD, LLC. All rights reserved. Used with permission.

48. Many doctors question the value of the postcoital test to check for infertility. It is not done very often.

49. The information to this point references the work of Dr Janice L. Andreyko, Northern California Fertility Medical Center, Recurrent Miscarriage, Updated September 21, 2012 http://www.ncfmc.com/recurrent-miscarriage.aspx.

50. Dr Marcus, Asherman's Syndrome, Details Asherman's Syndrome (AS) Last Updated June 19, 2011 10:03 p.m. GMT http://www.ivf-infertility.com.

51. A lot of people have this mutation and at this time there is no "standard of care" protocol for dealing with the presence of the gene mutation and recurrent pregnancy loss. The information about MTHFR is drawn from the work of Dr. Stephen Wells, Obstetrics, Gynecology, Fertility Walnut Creek, CA. Accessed September 2012, MTHFR & Recurrent Pregnancy Loss, http://stephenwellsmd.com/mthfr.htm.

52. Some centers will not take you as a patient if you and your partner smoke.

53. This is the average. It can fall anywhere from 10 to 17 days long.

54. This condition could cause miscarriage, but your specialist usually has newly pregnant women on progesterone to which will help the condition.

55. Please refer to the previous discussion of the female reproductive system we discussed the various hormones needed for conception, where they are located, and their job in the menstrual cycle.

56. Even so, some women have been known to conceive even while nursing.

57. Galactorrhea is another condition that occurs with high prolactin levels in the blood and is usually caused by the tumors on the pituitary gland. It causes milk production without being pregnant or recently having a child. This condition can also occur in men http://sharedjourney.com/define/prolactin.html.

58. Go to this site and it will calculate your BMI in standard measure or metric system: www.nhlbisupport.com/bmi/. Simply put your height in as number of feet and inches then put your weight and hit calculate. The site will give you your BMI and give their values for normal, overweight and obese.

59. Two-thirds of patients who underwent laparoscopic examination showed evidence of previous PID and the women were unaware of it.

60. http://www.cdc.gov/std/pid/stdfact-pid.htm.

61. Kathleen Cahill Allison, American Medical Association, *Complete Guide to Women's Health*, "Polycystic Ovarian Disease," Random House, New York, p227.

62. Ref: http://www.infertilityspecialist.com/articles/polycystic-ovarian-syndrome-and-insulin-resistance.html , (Endocrinol & Metab Clin; 28(2), 6/99, p350.

63. Endometriosis can be mild, moderate or severe for some women.

64. Karen J Carlson MD, Stephanie A. Eisenstat MD, Terra Zipo-

ryn Ph.D.: *The New Harvard Guide to Women's Heath,* "Endometriosis," pp218-221, 450-451.

65. http://en.wikipedia.org/wiki/Uterine_septum

66. Susan M Lark MD, *Celestial Arts,* "Fibroid Tumors and Endometriosis," 1995, pp7-15.

67. Dr. Charles W. Monteith,Medical Director, Chapel Hill Tubal Reversal Center, Raleigh, NC 27609, http://www.tubal-reversal. net/blog/2011/tubal-ligation-reversal/reasons-for-a-blocked-fallopian-tube.html.

68. http://www.cdc.gov/vaccinesafety/vaccines/HPV/Index.html.

69. Ibid. Recent research on the vaccine Gardasil has indicated that there have been some deaths associated with this vaccine. The subject of vaccines is very controversial and keep in mind when a drug comes out and is new there is a chance of seeing side effects. VAERS has reported over 20,000 cases of side effects from the vaccine. HPV are a group of more than 150 related DNA viruses that cause cervical cancer. More than 40 of these viruses are passed on through sexually transmitted disease and small amounts are transmitted non -sexually. The vaccination has shown a decrease in the HPV virus from two of these types, so women still have to have regular PAP screenings. I can't conscientiously mention the vaccination without stating the findings of the side effects and deaths. If you are at all considering the vaccine, please do your homework first. The best protection against any STD is abstinence, but a safer alternative is protection-using condoms.
70. http://www.cdc.gov/std/hpv/stdfact-hpv.htm.

71. If you bring a lap top to look up a movie, be aware some

centers may block certain web sites and that you are in there to collect and not watch a full length movie.

72. A horse's normal volume for an ejaculate is around 40 mls, just to give you and idea of volume.

73. 3rd Edition; "Morphology," 4th Edition.

74. Modifying certain behaviors can improve a man's fertility and should be considered when a couple is trying to achieve pregnancy.

75. Male factor is a term used for any infertility problems that have to do with the male partner.

76. "Shared Journey, Your Path to Fertility: Antisperm Antibodies: Accessed," October 12, 2012, http://www.sharedjourney. com/define/asperm.html

77. Dr. Mark Perole, Georgia Reproductive Specialist, *Miracle Babies*, "When Sperm Meets Egg-Sperm Interaction," http:// www.ivf.com/ch15mb.html.

78. Dr. Malpani, Malpani Infertility Clinic, Bombay India; http:// www.drmalpani.com/book/chapter7.html, low sperm count.

79. This section relies heavily on the work of Linda J. Vorvick, MD, Medical Director, MEDEX Northwest Division of Physician Assistant Studies, University of Washington, School of Medicine; Scott Miller, MD, Urologist in private practice in Atlanta, Georgia. Also reviewed by David Zieve, MD, MHA, Medical Director, A.D.A.M., Inc. *Medline Plus*, "Undescended Testicle," Updated 9/16/11, http://www.nlm.nih.gov/medlineplus/ency/ article/000973.htm.

80. Ref: wernermd.com/varicocele. This is an excellent site for male infertility.

81. http://www.auanet.org/content/press/press_releases/article.cfm?articleNo=69.

82. Dr Aniruddha Malpani, MD, Malpani Infertility Clinic, Jamuna Sagar, SBS Road, Colaba, Bombay 400 005, India; http://www.drmalpani.com/male-infertility.htm.

83. Congenital meaning that the baby is born with this condition.

84. There are three types of sperm extraction. Whichever extraction procedure is performed depends upon the type of blockage or damage. This is a surgical procedure where a sample of tissue is taken where the physician feels that there is sperm present. Dr. Aniruddha Malpani, MD, Malpani Infertility Clinic, Jamuna Sagar, SBS Road, Colaba, Bombay 400 005, India, http://www.drmalpani.com/book/chapter4b.html.

85. Dr. Samuel Marcus, FRCS FRCOG, "Surgical sperm retrieval" (PESA and TESA); http://www.ivf-infertility.com/ivf/pesa.php. Updated January 2, 2012.

86. Wikipedia: Klinefelters syndrome

87. *MedlinePlus* http://www.nlm.nih.gov/medlineplus/ency/article/000411.htm, updated 5/8/12.

88. *Shared Journey, Your Path to Fertility*, "Prolactin in Men," http://www.sharedjourney.com/malediagnosis/prolactin.html.

89. Ng/dl is a standards of measure in the blood which is nano-grams /deciliters. All lab results are resulted with a standard of measurement, each test has it's own measurement i.e. glucose is reported as mg/dl.

90. It is estimated that low testosterone affects more than 13 million men in the U.S.

91. Abraham Harvey Kryger, MD,DMD, *A Women's Guide to Men 's Health,* RDR Books, Berkely , Muskegon' "Low testoter-one," pp186, 190-191, 250.

92. This section is drawn largely from Stanton C. Honig M.D., "Public Enemy #1 for Male Fertility: Anabolic Steroids," University of Connecticut School of Medicine; Staff Physician, Yale New Haven Hospital; Hospital of St. Raphael, Urology Center, New Haven Hospital.

93. Dr. Stephen Lazarou, Urologist, Newton Wellesley Hospital, Newton, Massachusetts.

94. Ref: Dr. Stanley Ducharme Ph.D., *Physical Disability and Rehabilitation,* "Sex Therapy and Relationship," Boston Massachusetts, accessed September 10, 2012,http://www.stanley-ducharme.com/resources/anxiety.htm. Used with permission.

95. Such as Viagra.

96. http://en.wikipedia.org/wiki/erectile_dysfunction.
97. Stanley Ducharme, Ph.D. "Ejaculation Problems: Too Fast, Too Slow or Not at All? Early and Delayed Ejaculation: Psychological Considerations," November 29, 2003http://www.bumc.bu.edu/sexualmedicine/informationsessions/ejaculation-prob-lems-too-fast-too-slow-or-not-at-all/.

98. Scott Roseff, MD, FACOG, Jupiter, FL, http://www.repro-endo.com/html/female-infertility.html : South Florida Institute for Reproductive Medicine.

99. Dr. Aniruddha Malpani, MD, http://www.drmalpani.com/amh.htm, Malpani Infertility Clinic, Jamuna Sagar, SBS Road, Colaba, Bombay 400 005, India.

100. This is prescribed by a physician and the patient must be closely monitored.

101. Livestrong: http://www.livestrong.com/article/100961-dhea-female-fertility/#ixzz1gWx5yfSE; visited 4/27/13.

102. Oxidative stress is stress on the body that is caused by cumulative damage of free radicals that is not neutralized by antioxidants is a main contributor to sperm DNA fragmentation. The body needs oxygen. This, in combination with what we eat, burns to make energy for the body. There is a controlled metabolic process, which unfortunately produces dangerous by-products, including free radicals. These free radicals cause havoc on other cells in the body and affect the testicles in sperm production.

103. Sram, R.J., Benes, I., Binkova, B., Dejmek, J., Horstman, D., Kotesovec, F., Otto, D., Perreault, S.D., Rubes, J. & Selevan, S.G. et al. (1996) Teplice program -- "The impact of air pollution on human health," *Environ Health Perspective*, vol 104, 699-714.
104. Sepaniak, S., Forges, T. & Monnier-Barbarino, P. (2006) "Cigarette smoking and fertility in women and men," *Gynecol Obstet Fertil*, vol 34, 945-9; Martin, J. A., Hamilton, B. E., Sutton, P. D., et al (2005) Births: final data for 2004. Natl. Vital Stat. Rep. 54, 1–116.

105. Wryobek, A.J., Eskenazi, B., Young, S., Arnheim, N., Tiemann-Boege, I., Jabs, E.W., Glaser, R.L., Pearson, F.S. & Evenson, D.P. (2006) Advancing age has differential effects on DNA damage, chromatin integrity, gene mutations, and aneuploidies in sperm. *Proc Natl Acad Sci*, vol 103, 9601-6.

106. Virro, M.R., Larson-Cook, K.L. & Evenson, D.P. (2004) Sperm chromatin structure assay (SCSA®) related to blastocyst rate, pregnancy rate and spontaneous abortion in IVF and ICSI cycles. *Fertility and Sterility*, vol 81, 1289-1295.

107. Donald Evenson, Ph.D, HCLD,SCSA; Diagnostics, Inc. https://www.scsadiagnostics.com/contact company, visited 4/27/2013 (19).

108. Karen N. Peart, Yale University, *Yale News*; "Yale Researchers Develop Test to Identify 'Best' Sperm," May 20, 2010; http://news.yale.edu/2010/05/20/yale-researchers-develop-test-identify-best-sperm.

109. Ibid., Peart.

110. The hysteroscopy looks at the uterine lining and the Mary's test came back with fibroids. Fibroids are muscular tumors that can grow in the wall of the uterus and they can cause pain and increased bleeding during the menstrual cycle or in between the menstrual cycles. The HSG is the test that looks for blocked fallopian tubes and in Mary's case her tubes were fine, so in this case, the test came back normal.

111. A cycle is equal to one month. One patient could take three to four cycles (months) before she is successful.

112. If you look on-line at the different infertility clinics each center keeps track of there own IUI success. The National Average for ART cycles has to do more with IVF cycles.

113. It's very important to drink a lot of water when you are having your blood drawn, especially on a daily basis.

114. See Chapter 9 "Female Testing." In this chapter the RE performed the Clomid challenge test to check ovarian reserve.

115. Some of the medications now come in a pen with which you dial-up the amount of medication and add a sterile needle to the top of the pen.

116. There might be as many as 20 or more patients there for the same thing when you are waiting for your ultrasound and blood draw. A patient mentioned to me that when she saw the number of people in the waiting room, it made her feel better to realize there are other women in the same boat.

117. This section draws heavily upon the work of Dr. Aniruddha Malpani, MD, http://www.drmalpani.com/injections.htm , Malpani Infertility Clinic, Jamuna Sagar, SBS Road, Colaba, Bombay 400 005, India.

118. The following sites have videos to help with preparation and administering medications: Freedom MedTEACH; http://healthcare.walgreens.com/images/pdfs/pharmacy/Fertility_Education_v6.0_InjectionTrainingGuide.pdf.
119. As mentioned in Chapter 8, the nurses will have you test your ovulation the same time of the day, either in the morning or early afternoon, so that you can consult him/her that same day, before 5:00 p.m. If the results are positive for ovulation, the nurses will tell you to have your partner go to the center to pro-

duce a specimen or drop off the specimen that next morning.

120. You are not use to seeing a semen specimen in a collection cup and when it's first ejaculated it will be in one corner of the cup and it needs to liquefy which takes about 20 minutes. After it liquefies the sample will cover the bottom of the cup. You'll see the difference if you are delivering the specimen. And if for some reason the volume is low, the lab can add some media to the specimen, which will help the volume.

121. This refers to the number of sperm and volume of the sample. This is where the days abstinence is important; if a patient had intercourse the evening before and gave a sample the next morning, then the sample will have a lower count and less volume.

122. I know it can be a little embarrassing but it happens to all patients and the ultrasound technicians understand and help you keep everything covered; you are under a sheet the complete time.

123. FSH medications cause some patients to develop cysts on their ovaries, which usually disappear on their own after a month without medications.

124. This may or may not cover the medications. Each insurance company has different stipulations.

125. Not everyone needs over 20 eggs to be able to freeze embryos but each center has a certain protocol on number and quality of embryos that are produced to be able to freeze.

126. This section draws heavily from the work of Dr. Aniruddha Malpani, MD, http://www.drmalpani.com/book/chapter23.Mal-

pani Infertility Clinic, Jamuna Sagar, SBS Road, Colaba, Bombay 400 005, India.

127. Over stimulation of the ovaries (producing a lot of follicles) could lead to significant discomfort for the woman and in rare cases, can result in ovarian hyperstimulation syndrome, OHSS.

128. If three or fewer follicles are produced the IVF cycle may be cancelled.

129. This is a short protocol is also used for patients who had or are expected to have a low response to ovarian stimulation because of DOR (Diminished Ovarian Reserve) based on FSH levels.

130. Sandy Vance, RN , Flare Protocol.

131. This enables the RE to identify where she is at any given point in the cycle. This is important because the best place to start the IVF protocol is after the patient ovulates. The medication given will take over the body's cycle to stimulate the ovaries to produce many follicles and prevent premature ovulation.

132. Some centers put the patient on birth control pills at the start of each cycle so this is not an issue.

133. Samuel Marcus FRCS FRCOG,http://www.ivf-infertility.com-egg collection for IVF; Updated March 3, 2013.

134. I would ask my patients, "How did the retrieval go?" The majority of them said they didn't feel a thing, while others said who had a lot follicles (over 20) removed said that they were sore afterwards.

135. Other aspects of the microscopic appearance of the embryos are also noted including the presence of vacuoles, granularity, and thickness of the outer shell (or zona pellucida) of the embryo.

136. Arizona Center for Fertility Studies, Dr. Jay S. Nemiro, M.D. http://www.acfs2000.com/ivfservices/ivf-gradingIVFembryos. html.

137. The United Kingdom recently applied strict guidelines to the IVF procedure limiting the number of embryos transferred to women under 40 to two, and no more than three embryos for women over 40.

138. A good number of patients have several embryos left over from a single IVF cycle. If the embryos are of high quality, the couple can freeze the embryos for future cycles. When the couple is ready for another cycle they can do a "frozen cycle." This is less costly and safer for the female in that she doesn't have to start another round of injections to do a full stimulation cycle and the surgical procedure for retrieval is avoided. She will just take the medications needed to get the uterus ready for implantation with the embryos.

139. *Shared Journey – Your Path to Fertility*, "Assisted Hatching," www.sharedjourney.com/articles/ah.html; viewed June 23, 2013.

140. Also referred to as a "2WW" (two-week waiting).

141. When blood is drawn, the HCG renders a quantitative test, which gives a result as a measurable number; the urine pregnancy test is qualitative and gives only a positive or negative result. The RE can tell by the quantitative HCG result how the pregnancy is progressing normally or not.

142. I have had some patients come in for their second blood draw and ask me if the high HCG result from the first time suggested the presence of multiple embryos. I've seen high levels with multiple pregnancies but I've also seen it for a single pregnancy.

143. This section draws heavily upon: http://www.fertility-docs.com/PGD.phtml Medical Director Dr. Jeffrey M. Steinberg. The Fertility Institutes, 16030 Ventura Blvd. #404, Encino, CA 91436

144. PGD does not test for all chromosomal abnormalities and should not be substituted for mid-trimester genetic ultrasound evaluation and amniocentesis or chorionic villi sampling. PGD has likewise shown that in some instances repeated IVF failure could be caused by the sperm. There could be subtle genetic problems with the sperm that may explain why IVF cycles fail despite using PGD normal embryos.

145. At this time PGD is not recommended as a standard of practice for every IVF cycle. Couples should discuss with their doctors whether PGD is worth pursuing. Also, check with your specialist to confirm that the PGD testing is done at your center and see if they are looking at all chromosomes. Some testing looks only at one half of the number of chromosomes. Doctors make decisions on a case-by-case basis.

146. *Oxford Journals*, "Human Reproduction Multiple-birth Risk Associated with IVF and Extended Embryo Culture;" USA, 2001,

D.M. Kissin1,3, L.A. Schieve 2 and M.A. Reynolds 2, http://hum-rep.oxfordjournals.org/content/20/8/2215.full Hum. Reprod. (August 2005) 20(8): 2215-2223 first published online April 14, 2005.

147. Ibid., Kissin, Schieve, Reynolds.

148. Monozygote twins occur when one egg splits to form two embryos (identical twins) sharing one placenta.

149. *Reproduction, The Journal of the Society for Reproduction and Fertility,* "Monozygotic twinning associated with assisted reproductive technologies," a review: K I Aston1,23C M Peterson 4 and D T Carrell, 2,3,4 http://www.reproduction-online.org/ Received 14 May 2008 Revision, requested 13 June 2008. Accepted 23 June 2008 © 2008 Society for Reproduction and Fertility.

150. European Society of Human Reproduction and Embryology, Doctors issue alert over spontaneous natural conception while undergoing IVF, 2001 http://www.eurekalert.org/pub_releases/2001-10/esfh-dia102101.php. Public release date : 25-OCT-2001; Concurrent Conception last visited 11/25/12.

151. Dr. Marcus | : IVF-Infertility.com Last Updated May 29, 2013 3:23 p.m. GMT Ovarian hyperstimulation syndrome (OHSS)

152. Ibid., Marcus.

153. Ibid., Marcus.

154. http://fcionline.com/fertility-patients/consent-forms/OHSInstructions.pdf; fcipatientservices@integramed.com

155. Dr. Marcus | : IVF-Infertility.com Last Updated May 29, 2013

3:23 p.m. GMT Ovarian hyperstimulation syndrome (OHSS).

156. Dr. Marcus | Updated July 11, 2014 http://www.ivf-infertility. com/infertility/miscarriage.php.

157. Reprod Biomed Online. 2010 Feb;20(2):191-200. Epub 2009 Nov 26. http://www.ncbi.nlm.nih.gov/pubmed/20113957; "Miscarriage risk for IVF pregnancies in poor responders to ovarian hyperstimulation,"Haadsma ML, Groen H, Mooij TM, Burger CW, Broekmans FJ, Lambalk CB, Leeuwen FE, Hoek A; OMEGA Project Group.

158. Refer to the section on DFI in Chapter 14, p. 189.

159. It may be possible that she qualifies to use a new technique called preimplantation genetic diagnosis (PGD), which may reduce your risk of miscarriage in an IVF pregnancy particularly if there is a history of miscarriages before treatment.

160. UCSF Medical Center, FAQ Intracytoplasmic Sperm Injection, http://www.ucsfhealth.org/education/intracytoplasmic_ sperm_injection/; the risk of having a chromosomal abnormality like Down Syndrome is not increased with ICSI but increases with maternal age.

161. http://www.ucsfhealth.org/education/intracytoplasmic_ sperm_injection/.

162. http://www.sharedjourney.com/forums/andrology_embry-ology/assisted_hatching/.

163. *Women's Health, Health Information and More*, "IVF and Ectopic Pregnancy," http://www.womens-health.co.uk/IVF-ecto-pic-pregnancy.htm. Lasted visited 11/25/12.

164. Health statistics show that approximately one percent of all pregnancies is ectopic.

165. *Women's Health, Health Information and More*, "IVF and Ectopic Pregnancy," http://www.womens-health.co.uk/IVF-ectopic-pregnancy.htm. Lasted visited 11/25/ 12. Infertile patients have an increased risk of ectopic for unclear reasons. It could be because of a subtle tubal damage or blockage possible due to STDs (Sexually Transmitted Diseases).

166. Dr Aniruddha Malpani, MD, http://www.drmalpani.com/embryologist.htm, "IVF and Ectopic Preganancy," Malpani Infertility Clinic, Jamuna Sagar, SBS Road, Colaba, Bombay 400 005, India.

167. Ibid., Malpani.

168. Ibid., Malpani.

169. Ibid., Malpani.

170. Molar Pregnancy, MemeBridge 1550 Larimer St. #222, Denver, CO. 80202 http://www.molarpregnancy.net/, last accessed January 3, 2012.

171. Ibid., Molar Pregnancy.

172. The blood HCG levels that are drawn when you are first pregnant should rise in a certain manner which tells the specialist that everything is fine and you have a good pregnancy. And getting that first ultrasound usually shows what you have for number of fetuses and if there are any problems.

173. Ibid., Molar Pregnancy.

174. Ibid, Molar Pregnancy..

175. This section is adapted from ESHRE 2014 Meeting Abstract details; Submitter: Prof. Dr. Bert Scoccia, B. Scoccia1, K. Moghissi2, C. Westhoff3, S. Niwa4, D. Ruggieri5, B. Trabert6, E. Lamb7, L. Brinton6.; University of Illinois at Chicago, Obstetrics and Gynecology, Chicago IL, U.S.A.; Wayne State University, Obstetrics and Gynecology, Detroit MI, U.S.A.; Columbia University, Obstetrics and Gynecology, New York NY, U.S.A.. Westat Inc., Rockville MD, U.S.A.; IMS Inc., Rockville MD, U.S.A.; National Cancer Institute, Division of Cancer Epidemiology and Genetics, Bethesda MD, U.S.A.; Stanford University, Department of Obstetrics and Gynecology, Stanford CA, U.S.A.. Long-term relationship of ovulation-stimulating drugs to breast and gynecologic cancers; European Society of Human Reproduction and Embryology, 30 th Annual Meeting of ESHRE 2014, Munich Germany, June 2014, Session 17, page 4, O-06.

176. She would have blood work done and some ultrasounds to make sure the uterine lining is thickening.

177. Shady Grove Fertility, www.shadygrovefertility.com/newsletter/frozen-embryo-transfer-additional-treatement.

178. Vitrification (from Latin *vitreum,* "glass" via French vitrifier) is the transformation of a substance into a glass. Usually, it is achieved by rapidly cooling a liquid through the glass transition. Certain chemical reactions also result in glasses. An important application is the vitrification of an antifreeze-like liquid in cryopreservation (Wikipedia).

179. EVMS Medical Group Dr. Sergio Oehninger| EVMS Jones Institute for Reproductive Medicine, 601 Colley Avenue, Norfolk, VA 23507 | www.jonesInstitute.org.

180. EMVS. Fertil Steril. 2010 Jan;93(1):109-15. doi: 10.1016/j. fertnstert.2008.09.084. Epub 2008 Nov 21., Riggs R1, Mayer J, Dowling-Lacey D, Chi TF, Jones E, Oehninger S.

181. Ibid., Shady Grove Fertility.

182. That could include helping train the staff on techniques like ICSI or Assisted Hatching.

183. "The Maybe - Baby Dilemma," *Boston Globe Magazine*, November 22, 2009, p 22.

184. The nature of embryos remains controversial, politically, morally and religiously. At the core of the issue is the question of whether or not an embryo is a "life." This is an ongoing question and patients need to be aware of their own convictions about it before entering this difficult arena.

185. Ibid., "The Maybe - Baby Dilemma."

186. Lyerly A.D. & Faden R.R. "Embryonic stem cells. Willingness to donate frozen embryos for stem cell research," *Science* 317, 46–7 (2007).

187. "The Maybe - Baby Dilemma," *Boston Globe Magazine*, November 22, 2009, p 29.

188. Nightlight Christian Adoptions- http://www.nightlight.org; Pregnancy using donated embryos is sometimes called "embryo adoption." However, since the intended mother carries the pregnancy and gives birth, and there are no legal challenges to parental rights, the use of the term "embryo adoption" is not accurate. This could be a very viable program for some couples and it's away of using some of the extra embryos.

189. http://en.wikipedia.org/wiki/Nadya_Suleman.

190. "'Octomom' doctor loses California medical license," *Reuters*, Alex Dobuzinskis; Los Angeles,Wednesday June 1 2011. http://www.reuters.com/article/2011/06/01/us-octomom-idUSTR E7507TL20110601?feedType=RSS.

191. Shady Grove Fertility, Dr Eric Levens MD , Annadale, VA.

192. http://abcnews.go.com/Health/Politics/story?id=7023990 However, prior to this, embryo use for stem-cell research was limited by law, so few labs have been in the position to receive donations.

193. In addition to four years of training in obstetrics and gynecology, the MFM specialist has received two to three years of additional education in the diagnosis and treatment disorders of the mother and fetus.

194. This information is taken from http://laboratories.sequenom.com/maternit21plus/maternit21-plus-knowing-about-your-pregnancy.

195. Sequenom Laboratories, 3595 John Hopkins Court, San Diego, CA 92121, the MaterniT21-Plus test, http://laboratories.sequenom.com/maternit21plus/maternit21-plus-knowing-about-your-pregnancy.

196. For example, one clinic thatI am aware of marks age 43 years as the stopping point.

197. I had some patients after age 43 go to different centers that would do IVF and the couples were successful. Unfortunately,

there are a small percentage of patients that may never get pregnant.

198. Some women who have undergone several unsuccessful IVFs may experience a build up of scar tissue that can cause miscarriages or make it otherwise difficult to carry the baby to term. If this is the case, the patient may benefit from looking into a surrogate carrier, since, in this case, the surrogate carries the biological embryo of the client. Some women are fortunate and can have a sister or relative be the surrogate. Surrogates are usually women who have no problems carrying a baby and who love being pregnant. I knew of a woman that carried the embryo for her sister and brother-in-law. All went well and the sister delivered this couple a beautiful baby.

199. Religion plays into it only if there is a genetic component; for example if recipients are Jewish, there are some Jewish genetic diseases, which, if concerned, may suggest that the donor and recipient need to be tested.

200. Some programs do have deals to help patients cut the costs.

201. This particular program is from Shady Grove Fertility Center. (http://www.shadygrovefertility.com). There may be some differences in egg donor programs.

202. Information in this section comes from Shady Grove Fertility, located DC, MD, VA and PA. "About Our Donors," etc., last accessed January 31, 2013, http://www.shadygrovefertility.com/about-our-donors.

203. Shady Grove Fertility, located DC, MD, VA and PA. About Our Donors, last accessed January 31, 2013, http://www.shadygrovefertility.com/about-our-donors.

204. A baby was born in London from sperm that was frozen for 21 years. The father's sperm was frozen because of testicular cancer. bbc.co.uk.2004:25 May, *Guardian* 2004:25 May 2004.

205. Dr. Kirsty Horsey, "Progress Educational Trust Frozen Sperm as Good as Fresh," May 18 2004, *BioNews*, London.

206. Dr. Aniruddha Malpani, MD, http://www.drmalpani.com/eggfreezing.htm , Malpani Infertility Clinic, Jamuna Sagar, SBS Road, Colaba, Bombay 400 005, India.

207. Ibid., Malpani.

208. Ibid., Malpani

209. "Age and Elective Egg Freezing: The Allure of Postponing Childbearing Waxes as Odds of a Successful Outcome Wane," October 18,2011, ASRM Office of Public Affairs Published in ASRM Press Release emailed asrm@asrm.org.

210. "Stop Time," Sarah Wildman, New York Best Doctors, http://nymag.com/nymetro/health/features/14719/.

211. Dr. Gauri Bhide is a Medical Oncologist. How to preserve fertility during Cancer Treatments?, Practicing Oncologist in Boston, MA, wonderful website for any questions that pertain to cancer http://gauribhide.squarespace.com/ Tuesday, April 17, 2012.

212. FDA regulations donors require the potential donor to be tested every six months for STDs.

213. Wikipedia http://en.wikipedia.org/wiki/Sperm_donation_laws_by_country.

214. Wikipedia http://en.wikipedia.org/wiki/Sperm_donation_laws_by_country.

215. Dr. Aniruddha Malpani, MD, http://www.drmalpani.com/book/chapter28.html, Malpani Infertility Clinic, Jamuna Sagar, SBS Road, Colaba, Bombay 400 005, India.

216. Ibid., Malpani.

217. This paragraph and the one before it came from Dr. Aniruddha Malpani, MD, http://www.drmalpani.com/book/chapter29htm.

218. RESOLVE: The National Infertility Association is a non-profit, charitable organization, who works to improve the lives of women and men living with infertility.

219. https://www.childwelfare.gov/pubs/f_adoptoption.cfm.

220. You can find their secure website at: ifrr-registry.org.

Index

www.ingramcontent.com/pod-product-compliance
Lightning Source LLC
Chambersburg PA
CBHW031230090426
42742CB00007B/134